ELEMENTARY SCIENCE OF FOOD

ELEMENTARY SCIENCE OF FOOD

By

E. M. Hildreth, M.Sc.

(late Headmaster, The High School, Worsborough Dale, Barnsley)

Revised by Elisabeth Norton, B.Sc., D.I.C.

MILLS & BOON (with Allman & Son) LIMITED
17-19 Foley Street, London W1A 1DR

Fourth (revised) impression 1959
Fifth impression 1961
Sixth (revised) impression 1962
Seventh (revised) impression 1963
Eighth impression 1965
Ninth (revised) impression 1968
Tenth impression 1970
Eleventh impression 1971
Twelfth (fully revised) impression 1971
Thirteenth (revised) impression 1975
Fourteenth (revised) impression 1977

ISBN 0 263 05710 0

Printed photolitho in Great Britain by
Ebenezer Baylis & Son Limited
The Trinity Press, Worcester, and London

Contents

Preface

This book is essentially a simplified version of "Foods and Nutrition" written by the late W. Munn Rankin in collaboration with the author of this volume. It embodies the author's long and extensive experience in teaching the subject in secondary schools and technical colleges, and has been kept up to date by frequent revisions.

While the field it covers is an extensive one, the method of treatment makes it suitable for use by teachers and pupils in all types of secondary school, to those taking the relevant GCE examinations at "O" and "A" levels, to women in technical colleges preparing for cookery examinations of the City and Guilds of London Institute and similar bodies, and to students in domestic science training colleges.

The author is greatly indebted to the late W. Munn Rankin for much help and advice and to Miss M. King for reading the proofs and making many valuable suggestions. Any writer of food must inevitably lean on the *Manual of Nutrition*, published by H. M. Stationery Office, and I am glad to acknowledge the value of this publication. This latest edition has been revised by Mrs Elisabeth Norton and her help also is greatly valued.

Sincere thanks are also tendered to those who have supplied illustrations, the sources of which are acknowledged in the captions.

Worsborough Dale
Barnsley

E.M.H.

Conversion of Inches to Millimetres

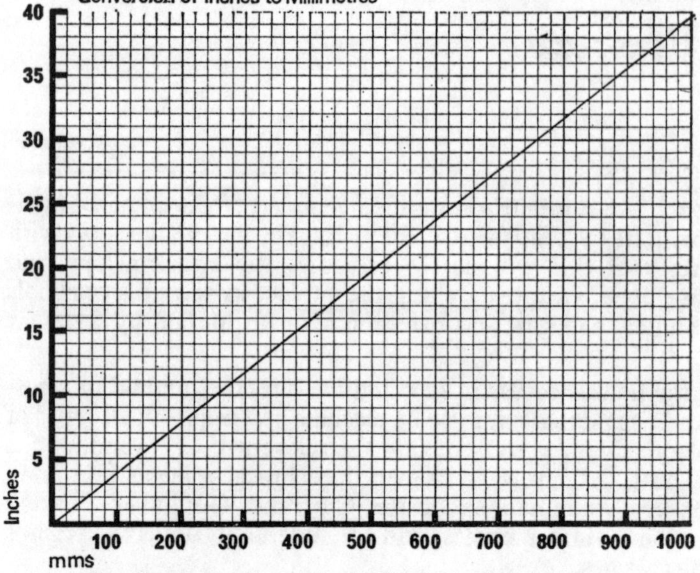

Conversion of International Units of Vitamin A to Micrograms

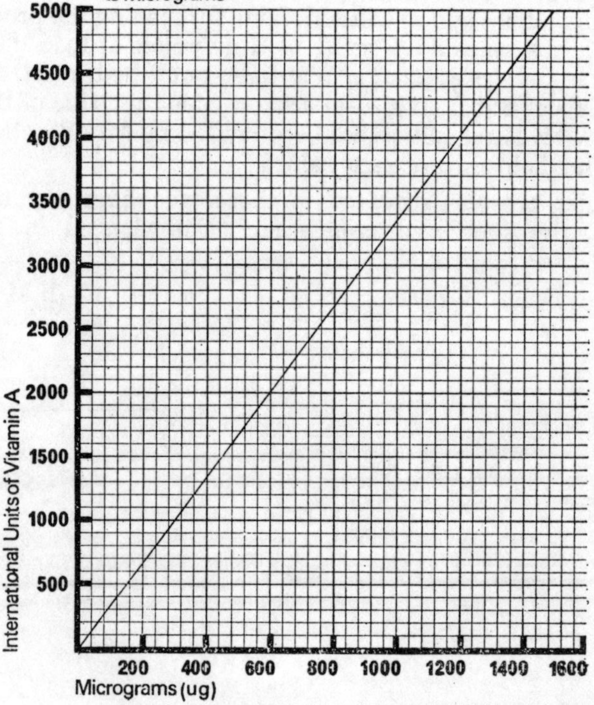

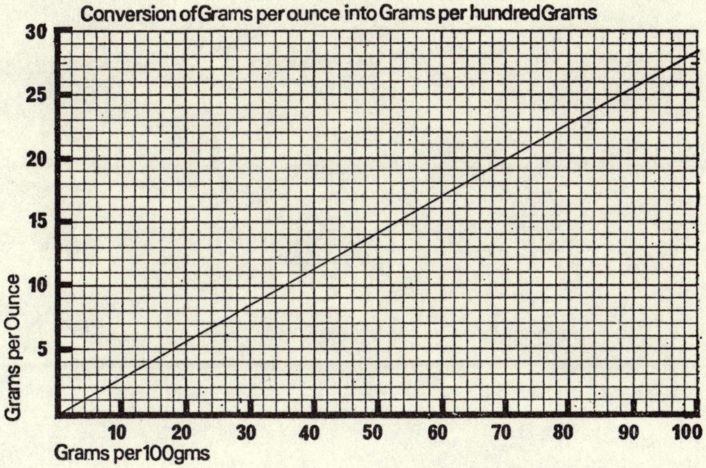

Conversion of Grams per ounce into Grams per hundred Grams
Grams per Ounce
30
25
20
15
10
5
10
20
30
40
50
60
70
80
90
100
Grams per 100gms

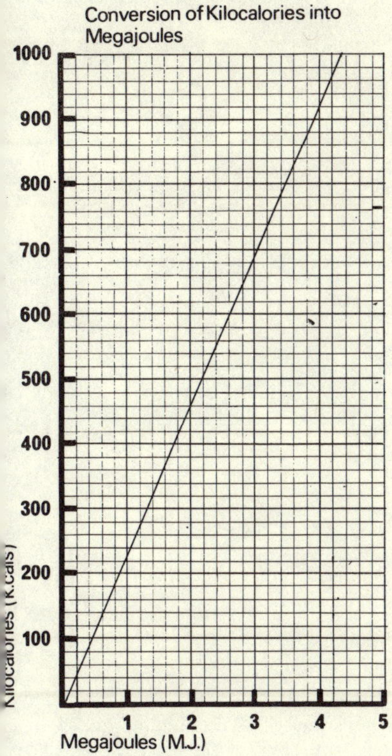

Conversion of Kilocalories into Megajoules
Kilocalories (K.Cals)
1000
900
800
700
600
500
400
300
200
100
1
2
3
4
5
Megajoules (M.J.)

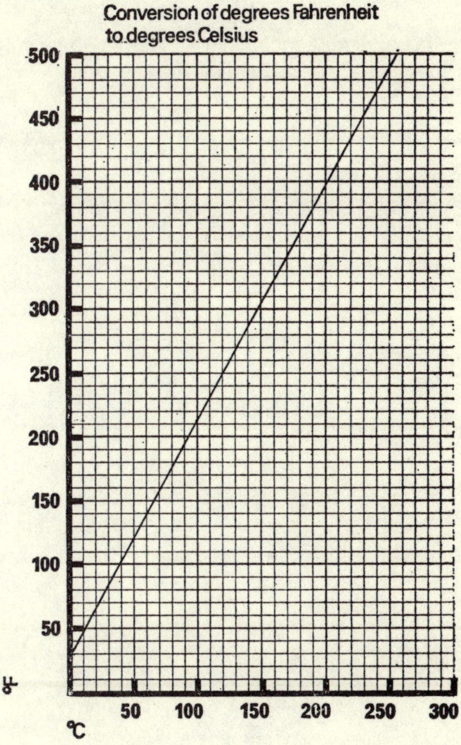

Conversion of degrees Fahrenheit to degrees Celsius
500
450
400
350
300
250
200
150
100
50
°F
50
100
150
200
250
300
°C

PART ONE

1 Why We Need Food

Like all other living things we need food to keep our bodies alive. This sounds very simple but is really very difficult because our bodies are extremely complicated organisms in which all sorts of processes are going on and all sorts of changes are taking place. For all these processes and changes which are involved in being alive, food is necessary in one way or another.

THE BODY AS A STOVE

We can think of our bodies as slow combustion stoves which give out heat all the time to the surrounding air and which must be supplied with suitable fuel at regular intervals. The fuel our bodies require is, of course, food. Whether we live near the North Pole or near the Equator, whether it is summer or winter, food keeps the temperature of our bodies steadily at blood heat, i.e. 36·9° C unless we are ill and have a "temperature."

THE BODY AS A MACHINE

Or, again, our bodies can be considered as machines which obtain their energy to work by burning food as fuel just as motor cars and aeroplanes burn petrol, and locomotives burn oil. Our muscles need energy to move our limbs when we walk, run, dig, lift and carry things or, in fact, whenever we are in any way physically active. All the many movements of our internal organs such as the beating of the heart and breathing, require energy which must be supplied by food.

THE BODY AS A STRUCTURE

Our bodies can also be considered as buildings which are being built up and kept in repair from the materials supplied by food just as ordinary buildings are built up and kept in repair by the use of bricks, stone, wood, cement and so on. When we are young we are steadily growing, putting on weight, increasing in height and generally building more and more material into our bodily structure. This goes on until we are fully grown adults and, in addition, throughout our lives, parts of our bodies are constantly being replaced.

THE BODY AS A CHEMICAL LABORATORY

Lastly, our bodies may be thought of as very busy chemical laboratories or workshops in which all sorts of complicated substances are being made out of the raw materials which go into them in the form of food. All these activities, and more, are those of ourselves as living organisms and all are dependent upon our getting not only enough food but food of the right kinds.

Summing up very briefly, the principal purposes for which we need food are:

1. To supply energy as a source of work and heat.
2. To supply building and repair materials.
3. To supply substances which are required for the chemical changes which take place in our bodies.

SOURCES OF FOOD

Green plants obtain their food from the carbon dioxide of the air which they take in through their leaves and from the water, with its dissolved mineral substances from the soil, which they obtain through their roots. The green colouring material in their leaves, which is called chlorophyll, enables green plants to absorb energy from the sun. This they use to convert the carbon dioxide, water and mineral salts into the substance of, say, grass, or an onion, or an oak tree. Some plants, known as *fungi*, such as mushrooms, moulds and yeasts, and also bacteria can live without sunshine but only by feeding upon the substance of green plants or animals.

Animals either feed upon green plants or prey upon other animals which have eaten plants. The first type are *herbivorous* animals, e.g., sheep, cattle and horses; the second type are *carnivorous*, e.g., lion, tiger and fox.

Human beings are both carnivorous and herbivorous, i.e. *omnivorous*, since they eat both animal and plant foods. There are, however, races of people who are almost entirely carnivorous, e.g., the Eskimo. Other races of mankind are almost entirely herbivorous or vegetarian, e.g., the Hindu, and there are people who from principle or choice are strict vegetarians. The majority of human beings, however, rely upon a mixed diet of animal and plant foods and there is no doubt that, when wisely chosen, such a mixed diet is best able to maintain good health for most people.

Because human beings use both animals and plants as sources of food there is an enormous variety of articles from which to choose. But it is now known that all such articles of food consist of some half dozen sorts of substances which are known as *nutrients*, each of which plays its special part in meeting one or other of the needs of our bodies. The nutrients are CARBOHYDRATES, FATS, PROTEINS, MINERALS, VITAMINS and WATER. Carbohydrates and fats supply energy for work and heat. Proteins, and some minerals, supply building and repair materials. Other minerals, and the vitamins, are needed for the chemical processes which go on in the body while water acts partly as a building material and partly as the medium for the transport of materials generally within the body.

The Nutrients

1. CARBOHYDRATES	The main supply of energy.
2. FATS	The chief subsidiary supply of energy.
3. PROTEINS	The building and repair substances. Also used to supply energy.
4. MINERALS	Some provide building materials; others are needed for chemical processes.
5. VITAMINS	Essential in small amounts for chemical processes.
6. WATER	A building material and a medium for the transport of materials generally, within the body.

In any well-balanced mixed diet all the nutrients are present in sufficient amount to maintain our bodies in good health. If the diet is lacking in one or other of the nutrients then our bodies will be ill-nourished and our health suffer accordingly.

GENERAL SOURCES OF NUTRIENTS

The carbohydrates are starches and sugars so that our main carbohydrate foods are such starchy foods as bread, potatoes and oatmeal, and such sugary foods as cane sugar, sweets, jam and syrup. Our chief fat foods are butter, margarine, cooking fats and oils, cheese, milk and meat. Proteins and minerals for body-building are provided in milk, eggs, meat, fish, cheese, pulses, cereals, nuts, and some vegetables. Minerals and vitamins for vital chemical processes in the body are supplied by such foods as milk, fruit, vegetables, eggs, bread, flour, cheese and fish. We can set out the main purposes of the nutrients as follows:

A. Nutrients and Foods Providing Energy
Carbohydrates: starch—bread, potatoes, oatmeal,
sugar—cane sugar, sweets, jam and syrup.
Fats: suet, dripping, butter, margarine, lard, cooking oils.

B. Nutrients and Foods Providing Building and Repair Materials
Proteins: milk, eggs, meat, fish, cheese, pulses, cereals and nuts.
Minerals: milk, eggs, meat, fish, cheese, pulses, cereals, nuts and some vegetables.

C. Nutrients and Foods Essential For Chemical Processes
Minerals: milk, fruit, vegetables, eggs, fat fish, bread and flour.
Vitamins: milk, cheese, eggs, meat, fish, butter, margarine, flour, and some vegetables and fruit.

A. Food as a Source of Energy (Work and Heat)

As we have already seen, life consists essentially of processes and operations which require energy. Green plants are able to utilise energy from the sun which they absorb with the help of the chlorophyll of their leaves. Animals and human beings are unable to do this. They can only obtain their energy at second hand either from plants or from other animals which have eaten plants. This locked-up energy is released by burning (or oxidation) by means of the oxygen which animals and human beings breathe into their lungs. This oxidation is exactly similar to burning in ordinary air except that it takes place very much more slowly and there is, of course, no flame. Just as carbohydrates (starch and sugar) and fats form carbon dioxide and water vapour when they are burnt in air, so they do in our bodies and these are the things we breathe out.

In both cases the same amounts of heat and energy are released and this is the heat and energy which was originally absorbed by green plants from sunlight.

So you see that the energy we use to work and move about and the heat that keeps us warm, are really the sun's heat and energy which come to us by way of the plants and animals we eat.

THE UNITS FOR THE MEASUREMENT OF ENERGY

Before we can consider how much food energy we require each day we must decide how this energy can be measured.

The simplest answer to this is that the food energy we take in and use up is most conveniently measured in terms of the heat that would be given out if all our food were burnt, i.e., oxidised, as in the body. That amount of heat equals exactly the sum of the energy which is converted into work and the waste energy given out as heat. We can only do any kind of physical work at the expense of energy. The more work we do, the more energy we require, which means we require more food containing energy. But it happens that most of the energy locked up in our food (about 85%) cannot be converted into work, but is reduced to the lowest form of energy, which is heat, and is liberated as heat.

The unit that has been used in the past to reckon the energy values of foods, and of fuels in general, is the kilocalorie (kcal) often referred to as the Calorie (Cal).

The kilocalorie is defined as the amount of heat needed to raise the temperature of one kilogramme of water by one degree Celsius.

However, with the adoption of the standard metric system, energy is measured in joules. A thousand kcal is equivalent to 4·186 million joules, or 4·186 megajoules (MJ). One megajoule may be defined as the amount of heat energy needed to raise the temperature of approximately 239 grammes of water by one degree Celsius. 1 kcal is approximately equivalent to 4·1 KJ.

It has been found that one gram of carbohydrate (as glucose) is absorbed and oxidised in the body to produce 3·75 kcal (or 0·0157 MJ). An average pure fat gives 9·3 kcal (or 0·039 MJ) per gramme. When a protein is used up in the body it is not completely oxidised and its heat output is at the rate of 4·1 kcal per gramme (or 0·0175 MJ per gramme).

Thus 1 g carbohydrate yields 3·75 kcal (approx. 4 kcal) or 0·0157 MJ.
1 g. Fat yields 9·3 kcal (approx. 9 kcal) or 0·039 MJ.
1 g. Protein yields 4·1 kcal (approx. 4 kcal) or 0·0175 MJ.

This means that fats provide more than twice the amount of energy provided by the same weight of carbohydrate or protein.

B

Fats are our most concentrated energy foods. Carbohydrates are less concentrated energy foods but are cheaper than fats while proteins are expensive and are really wasted as energy foods since their real purpose in the body is to supply material for growth and repair. Fats and carbohydrates are not body-builders.

Our main energy foods are bread, flour and other cereals, sugar and sugary foods (treacle, jam etc.), meat, visible fats (butter, margarine, suet, cooking oil, dripping) and dairy foods. Our main starchy vegetable is the potato. Articles of food such as bread, cakes, pastry, biscuits and suet pudding which are made from carbohydrates and fats are also, of course, energy foods. Pulses (such as peas, beans, lentils and soya) and dried fruits are also useful sources of energy.

Why We Require Energy

1. To maintain the normal temperature of the body.

2. To maintain the beating of the heart and circulation of the blood, breathing, and the many other movements of internal organs.

3. To maintain the chemical processes within the cells of the body as in secretion, excretion and respiration.

4. For all physical activity—sitting, standing, walking, running, playing games and for all kinds of manual and muscular work in the home, workshop, garden, field and so on.

The rate at which the basic processes go on in our body is called the *Basal Metabolic Rate.* These processes are those that are working all the time, that are basic to the living body and include:– the control of body temperature, the beating of the heart, the workings of the internal organs, and so on. Thus the basal metabolic rate is in effect the rate at which the body uses energy while we are at rest. As soon as physical work is done more energy is needed, and the harder the work the more energy will be used.

The basal metabolic rate is roughly proportional to the total surface area of the skin of a person; so the larger they are the higher their metabolic rate will be. In fact this is, of course, only an approximation and any one person's basal metabolic rate is likely to be slightly different from the average and can vary from time to time.

Factors effecting the basal metabolic rate include:—

1. **Age.** It varies with age, it increases from birth up till the age of about 25, and decreases from the age of about 35 onwards.

2. **Sex.** Women have a lower metabolic rate than men.
3. **Meal times.** The metabolic rate rises after one has eaten, which is one reason why it is not a good thing to have long intervals between meals.
4. **Level of Nutrition**. Starvation or prolonged under-nutrition causes a fall in the metabolic rate.
5. **Exercise.** Exercise causes a rise in the metabolic rate as well, of course, as using energy for the movement itself.
6. **Sleep.** Sleep causes a fall in the basal metabolic rate.
7. **Illness** and **emotional disturbances**. These can alter the metabolic rate.
8. **Drugs.** These can alter the basal metabolic rate.

If we accept that all these factors will affect the metabolic rate but that on average it is possible to arrive at a generalised figure for any one person, we are now in a position to consider their total energy requirements. These will be determined by their basal metabolic requirements **plus** the energy needed for their physical activities. The following table gives recommended energy requirements for people of various ages at different levels of physical activity. When using these tables we must always bear in mind the personal variations that may exist; we must also remember that the level of physical work is an overall one and that a short spell of hard digging will not entitle one to the kcal. intake of a very active person!

Daily Energy Intakes

Age	Occupation	Energy (kcal)	MJ
Children			
0–1 year		800	3·3
1–2		1,200	5·0
2–3		1,400	5·9
3–5		1,600	6·7
5–7		1,800	7·5
7–9		2,100	8·8
Boys			
9–12		2,500	10·5
12–15		2,800	11·7
15–18		3,000	12·6

Age	Occupation	Energy (kcal.)	MJ
Girls			
9–12		2,300	9·6
12–15		2,300	9·6
15–18		2,300	9·6
Men			
18–35	sedentary	2,700	11·3
	moderately active	3,000	12·6
	very active	3,600	15·1
35–65	sedentary	2,600	10·9
	moderately active	2,900	12·1
	very active	3,600	15·1
65–75	assuming sedentary	2,350	9·8
75–	life	2,100	8·8
Women			
18–55	most occupations	2,200	9·2
	very active	2,500	10·5
55–75	assuming sedentary	2,050	8·6
75–	life	1,900	8·0
Late Pregnancy		2,400	10·0
Lactation		2,700	11·3

Recommended by the Dept. of Health and Social Security (1969)

We may now proceed to calculate the energy values of diets. The average daily intake of a man is about 1·3 kg. This will contain about 368 g of carbohydrate, 141 g of fat and 85 g of protein, the remainder being made up of water, indigestible fibre residue and minute quantities of vitamins and minerals.

Nutrient	*Quantity g*	*kcal value per gramme*	*kcal*
Carbohydrate	368	3·75	368 × 3·75 = 1,380
Fat	141	9·3	141 × 9·3 = 1,311
Protein	85	4·1	85 × 4·1 = 348
			Total kcal = 2,939

Deducting 10% for wastage in cooking and from plates this would give approximately 2,636 kcalories per day.

Another example is given by the diet of a moderately active woman which consisted of 320 grammes of carbohydrate, 107 grammes of fat and 76 grammes of protein.

Nutrient	*Quantity* g	*kcal value per gramme*	*kilocalories*
Carbohydrate	320	3·75	320 × 3·75 = 1,200
Fat	107	9·3	107 × 9·3 = 995·1
Protein	76	4·1	76 × 4·1 = 311·6
			Total kcals per day = 2,506·7

or approximately 2,500 kilocalories per day.

The kcal value of a particular food can be calculated in a similar way. White bread contains 54·6 g carbohydrate, 1·7 g fat and 8·3 g protein per 100 g.

Nutrient	*Quantities* g/100 g	*kcal. value per gramme*	*kcal*
Carbohydrate	54·6 g	3·75	54·6 × 3·75 = 204·8
Fat	1·7 g	9·3	1·7 × 9·3 = 15·8
Protein	8·3 g	4·1	8·3 × 4·1 = 34
			Total kcal = 254·6

If, for any reason, we do not obtain our energy needs from our food we quickly feel hunger and, sooner or later, find that we become slimmer and less and less capable of hard work. People who need a large number of kcalories should eat increased amounts of the energy nutrients, i.e., fats and carbohydrates, and foods made from them such as bread, cakes, pastry, biscuits and puddings, but these quickly become fattening if eaten in excess of need.

B. Food as a Source of Building Materials (Proteins and Minerals)

We require food to supply material for the growth and repair of the tissues of the body. Our bodies are made up of millions and millions of microscopical units, the *cells*, which increase enormously in number as we pass from infancy to manhood or womanhood. The baby weighing a few kilogrammes at birth cannot grow and develop into the adult weighing twenty-five kilogrammes or more without obtaining considerable amounts of suitable building materials. In addition, throughout life, the cells are continually being reconstructed. All this growth and repair depends upon food and one type of nutrient in particular. This is *protein.* The cells of our bodies consist essentially of a substance called "*protoplasm.*" This has been well described as "the physical basis of life." It consists almost entirely of protein. Plants can form their own protein and protoplasm from carbon dioxide of the air, and from water with its dissolved mineral substances absorbed from the soil. Human beings and animals cannot do this. We, and animals generally, are dependent for our supply of protein upon plants or other animals which live on plants. It is indeed true in a very real sense that "All flesh is grass."

There are thousands of proteins, for no two species of plants or animals contain exactly the same proteins.

AMINO-ACIDS

Nevertheless, all proteins, no matter what their sources, are now known to be built up of a very small number of units or "building blocks." These are known as *amino-acids*. By linking together in elaborate chains, networks and foldings, these amino-acids build up the vast variety of plant and animal proteins. When we digest the proteins in our food they are broken down bit by bit into their constituent amino-acids. These pass into our system and are used to build up the various proteins of its cells and tissues. It is plain that unless we get in our food the amino-acids required to build up and repair our own particular proteins, then growth and repair, and indeed life itself, will cease. Any amino-acids which our bodies do not require for building and repair will be broken down and the energy they contain will be used by the body or set free as heat.

SOURCES OF PROTEIN

Our main protein or body-building foods are milk, eggs, meat, fish and cheese. Of these, milk and eggs are much the best and cheese is, perhaps, the cheapest of all body-building foods. It is natural that the proteins of animals should be the best for human beings since we are animals. Among plant foods, the pulses—peas, beans, lentils and soya; the cereals—wheat and oatmeal; and some nuts, contain very useful amounts of protein. As will be explained in the next chapter, they are not so valuable singly as are animal proteins. They are, however, useful supplementary sources of body-building material, especially when mixed.

BUILDING MINERALS

In addition to proteins the body requires certain minerals to help form part of its structure. Thus our bones and teeth are hardened and made rigid or "calcified" by being supplied with *calcium* and *phosphorus* from food. Milk is an excellent source of both ingredients.

The red corpuscles of the blood contain *haemoglobin* which absorbs oxygen from the air we breathe into our lungs and carries it in the circulation to every living cell in the body. There it helps in the release of energy from food substances also transported by the blood. An essential element in the haemoglobin is *iron*, which must, therefore, be supplied in our food. Lack of iron is very evident in anaemia or "bloodlessness."

Another element of use as a building material is *iodine*. This is needed by the thyroid glands which lie on either side of the wind-pipe towards the base of the neck. They manufacture a substance called *thyroxine* which contains iodine. Thyroxine is passed into the blood stream. Without thyroxine, physical and mental growth cannot proceed satisfactorily. One form of goitre is due to the low activity of the thyroid glands. Sea foods, iodised table salt and iodised sweets are excellent sources of iodine.

A summary of the best food sources of the minerals required for body-building is given below.

Minerals for Body-Building

Mineral	*Sources*
Calcium	Milk, cheese, egg yolk, oatmeal, watercress, "hard" water, flour.
Iron	Liver, meat, egg yolk, cocoa, sardines, oily fish, almonds, raisins, watercress, cabbage, flour.

Mineral	*Sources*
Phosphorus	Liver, kidney, egg yolk, meat, fish, milk, cheese.
Iodine	Sea foods (fish, shell fish), watercress, onions.

Fats for Body-Building

Fats are combined with the mineral phosphorus to form phosopholipids, and with proteins to form lipo-proteins, both of which are essential constituents of the cells of our bodies.

C. Food as a Source of Other Essential Chemical Constituents (Vitamins and Minerals)

Until about the year 1912 it was generally thought that if we ate sufficient fats and carbohydrates to supply the kilocalories we required and ate sufficient proteins for body-building and repair purposes, then our bodies would be getting everything necessary for life and health.

We now know that in addition to fats, carbohydrates and proteins, our bodies require certain substances called vitamins and some minerals. Without these *regulative or protective foods*, as they are often called, our bodies are unable to release the energy locked up in fats and carbohydrates and unable to lay down the necessary amino-acids to build up our tissues. We are unable to make full and proper use of the energy and body-building foods we eat and our health suffers—often very seriously. In fact, we are liable to suffer, in some degree, from such diseases as beri-beri, pellagra, scurvy and rickets. These are known as *deficiency diseases* because they are caused through a deficiency of one or other of the protective substances in the diet. In extreme cases these deficiency diseases are grave disorders which lead to much suffering and shortening of life. Beri-beri affects millions of rice eaters of the East. Pellagra is a scourge among the maize-eating negroes in the Southern States of U.S.A. Scurvy has killed more sailors than warfare and shipwreck combined. Rickets crippled and stunted thousands of children in the slums of our great towns during the last century.

SOURCES OF VITAMINS

The amounts of these substances our bodies require are very small indeed, and are measured in milligrammes or microgrammes per day, but this is no measure of their importance. These very small amounts are absolutely essential to our health and, in fact, to our very lives. We obtain them chiefly from *dairy foods* such as butter, margarine, eggs, cheese and milk; from *fruits*, particularly summer berry fruits, tomatoes and citrus fruits such as oranges, lemons and grapefruit; from *vegetables*, such as cabbage, cauliflower, Brussels sprouts, carrots and potatoes; from *meat* and *liver*; from *fat fish* such as herrings, salmon and sardines; and from *bread* and *flour*. In other words, our most important protective foods are dairy foods, fruits, vegetables, meat, fat fish and bread.

We can now summarise what we have learned in the form of a table.

Type of food	*Consists of*	*Common examples*
Energy	Fats and Carbohydrates	Butter, margarine, suet, lard, dripping and cooking oils. Cereals (wheat, rice, oatmeal). Sugar, treacle, syrup, jam. Potatoes. Pulses. Dried fruit. And of course, things made from these, e.g. bread, cakes, pastry, biscuits, suet pudding. Cheese. Bacon and ham.
Body-building	Proteins and Minerals	Milk, eggs, meat, fish and cheese. Supplemented by wheat flour, peas, beans, lentils, soya and nuts.
Regulative or "Protective"	Minerals and Vitamins	Milk, cream, butter, eggs, cheese, margarine. Summer berry fruits and foreign citrus fruits. Vegetables, particularly green vegetables, carrots, potatoes. Fat fish such as herrings, salmon and sardines. Liver, meat, bread, flour.

There are several points about this table which must be made clear. Firstly, it is purely an artificial table drawn up for our convenience. With the exception of a very few foods such as sugar, which is purely an energy food, foods do not exactly fit into our scheme. Bacon and ham, for example, are important energy foods but they also supply protein and even some protective material as well.

Secondly, some foods such as cheese, milk, eggs and fat fish appear in more than one group. This should show you how very valuable and important these particular foods are in our diet.

Thirdly, a complete diet will contain an adequate amount of each type of food. The ones most likely to be insufficient in amount are the body-building and protective foods because these are the most expensive. We must first make certain that these are included and then look to the energy foods. In planning our meals we should ask ourselves these questions:

1. Have I included body-building foods?
2. Have I included sources of vitamins and minerals?
3. Have I included sufficient energy foods to satisfy appetite?

Fourthly, we must realise that we can ring the changes among foods of the same type. We can substitute one body-building food for another body-building food; one energy food for another energy food. Meat can be replaced by fish, cheese or eggs. Potatoes can be replaced by bread. Butter can be replaced by vitaminised margarine. But one type of food cannot do the work of another type. Meat cannot be replaced by jam; cheese cannot be replaced by cake; milk cannot be replaced by tea.

Fifthly, all this does not mean that we have to be cranks, and faddy about our food. There is no need for us to be forever wondering whether we are getting the right number of kilocalories or enough protein, or this particular mineral or that particular vitamin. Not at all! It simply means that our daily diet should be made up from the following foods:

1. *Milk*. At least a pint for everyone daily, more for children and expectant and nursing mothers.
2. *Eggs, Cheese, Pulses*. At least three or four times per week.
3. *Meat, Fish or Poultry*. Once daily. Fish should preferably be fat fish such as herrings, salmon and sardines.
4. *Fruit*. Orange, grapefruit or tomato. At least once daily.
5. *Vegetables*. Two kinds daily in addition to potatoes, and including one salad or green vegetable.
6. *Fats*. Butter or margarine.
7. *Cereals*. Bread and oatmeal are the most valuable.
8. *Water*. About 1·4 litres of fluids daily, some of which should be in the form of water itself, i.e., not as tea, coffee or cocoa. Eat any other foods you like in order to satisfy your appetite.

If you look at the table again you will see that our body-building materials come from milk, eggs, meat, cheese and flour, with additions from pulses; many of our vitamins and minerals from milk, butter, eggs, cheese, fruit, flour, vegetables, meat and fat fish; and our energy requirements are supplied by bread, oatmeal, butter, margarine, cheese and potatoes. The additional foods we eat to please our palates or to satisfy our appetites, e.g., cakes, pastry, biscuits, puddings, jam, treacle, syrup, and sweets, etc., are mainly energy foods.

The study of how nutrients supply the body's needs for energy, growth and protection is known as *nutrition*. If the body does not receive enough of any one of the nutrients it suffers from *malnutrition*. If the body receives too little of all the nutrients it suffers from *under-nutrition* or, in extreme cases, *starvation*.

Millions of people in the poorer under-developed countries of the world, such as Africa, Asia and parts of Latin America, are suffering from malnutrition or under-nutrition. At the same time their populations are increasing much more rapidly than their food production. This is one of the most urgent problems facing the world today.

In this and other highly developed countries the problems are not usually the result of a shortage of food. In the main they result either from over-eating, or from a lack of adequate knowledge of the correct foods that should be eaten. Over-eating which causes people to be too fat is usually due to the inclusion of too many sweet and starchy foods. Lack of knowledge of the correct foods to include in the diet may, of course, also lead to a person being over-weight, but it may also lead to malnutrition, stunted growth and poor health.

2 Carbohydrates

Carbohydrates consist of carbon, hydrogen and oxygen. The hydrogen and oxygen are present in the same proportions as in water (H_2O); hence the name carbohydrate. With very few exceptions, carbohydrates are plant products formed from carbon dioxide and water with the help of energy from the sun absorbed by the chlorophyll of leaves. At first, very simple carbohydrates are formed. From these, plants build up more complicated substances such as the sugar we call glucose. Glucose, in its turn, is built up into more complicated sugars, such as cane sugar. Still further building-up, or synthesis, results in the formation of starch and cellulose.

When we digest carbohydrates, they are broken down by our digestive juices in the reverse direction until, finally, they become glucose again. This passes into our blood stream and thence into the living cells and tissues. There it is oxidised or burned to carbon dioxide and water by the oxygen we have breathed in and energy and heat are released. As pointed out in the previous chapter, this energy is the energy originally obtained by plants from sunlight.

The Building-up of Carbohydrates in Plants

Carbon dioxide + water + energy from sunlight →
carbohydrates + oxygen.

The Breaking-down of Carbohydrates in our Bodies

Carbohydrates + oxygen → carbon dioxide + water
+ energy for heat and work.

There are three kinds of carbohydrates:

(a) *Sugars* (b) *Starches* (c) *Cellulose*

SUGARS

Sugars are divided into *single sugars* (*monosaccharides*) such as glucose or grape sugar and fructose or fruit sugar, and *double sugars* (*disaccharides*) which are formed by linking together two single sugars. Examples of double sugars are sucrose (cane sugar and beet sugar), lactose (milk sugar) and maltose (malt sugar). They all have a sweet taste, easily dissolve in water and are easily digested.

Glucose is found naturally in ripe fruits, plant juices and honey and, among vegetables, the onion is particularly rich in it. Glucose is now manufactured on a large scale from starch and much used in the manufacture of cheap jams and sweets.

All carbohydrate foods digested and absorbed in the body are converted into glucose in the liver and pass into the blood where it is maintained at a very steady concentration. The pancreas secretes a substance known as *insulin* which enables us to convert blood sugar, as the glucose in our blood is called, into *glycogen* or "*animal starch.*" Some of this glycogen is made in the muscles where it can quickly be reconverted into glucose if it is needed by the muscle for fuel. Glycogen is also stored in the liver and there forms a small reserve store of carbohydrate. During a long spell of muscular activity the glycogen in the muscles is used up and the glycogen in the liver is reconverted to glucose and passes to the muscles to replenish them.

Persons who are unable to form sufficient insulin from the pancreas suffer from *diabetes* and the amount of glucose in the blood rises until the kidneys remove the excess and pass it into the urine. Some diabetic patients need to have injections of insulin to help them to bring down to normal the concentration of their blood sugar. Glucose is frequently given to invalids and convalescents as a readily available source of heat and energy.

Adrenalin, the hormone produced by the adrenal glands near the kidneys, controls the withdrawal of glucose from the liver and a consequent rise in the concentration of glucose in the blood, e.g., during anger or fear, so that there is an immediate supply for additional energy if this is needed.

If the body takes in more glucose than it can use or store as glycogen the excess is converted into fat which is laid down in various parts of the body as a reserve. This fat can be converted back into glucose and energy when necessary. Foods rich in carbohydrates, such as potatoes and bread, can thus be fattening foods if we habitually eat more of them than we require for energy purposes.

Fructose, or fruit sugar, is another single sugar similar to glucose and is usually found along with it in ripe fruits, plant juices and honey. It is the sweetest of all sugars.

Sucrose is the scientific name for the sugar obtained from sugar cane and sugar beet. It is a *double sugar* (*disaccharide*) made up of a combination of glucose and fructose. Besides being found in sugar cane and sugar beet it occurs in ripe fruits, honey, sugar maple, beetroot, parsnips, carrots and dried fruits such as dates, prunes, currants, raisins and sultanas.

The highly refined table sugar which we most commonly use is the purest food we eat. It consists entirely of sucrose. Like other carbohydrates it is converted into glucose during digestion in the intestines and is a readily available energy food. Its sweet taste makes many other foods more palatable.

Of course, sugar contains no protective or body-building material and, if eaten in excess, it takes the edge off our appetite so that we may eat less of more valuable foods. There is little doubt that in this country most children and many adults eat too much sugar and sugar-containing foods and that the consumption of sugar is increasing. Sugar and sweets are "empty" in the sense that kilocalories are the only things they supply. In addition, readily fermented carbohydrates, such as sugar, in contact with the teeth tend to encourage tooth decay. Not too much and not too often is good advice so far as sugar and sweets are concerned. To have a "sweet tooth" is not an indication of wise eating.

Saccharin, which is often used as a sugar substitute, has no connection with sugar in spite of its sweet taste. It is an artificially prepared chemical substance and has no food value whatever. It passes through the body unchanged.

Lactose (milk sugar) is similar to sucrose but not so sweet. Unlike sucrose, it is an animal product present in all types of milk. It is formed from glucose and galactose.

Maltose (malt sugar) is the sugar formed from starch when barley grains are made into malt by germination. It is formed from glucose.

STARCH

Unlike the sugars, starch is not sweet and is insoluble in cold water. It is made up of numerous glucose units linked together as in a long chain. Hence it is called a *polysaccharide*. It is in the form of insoluble starch that most plants store up the carbohydrate they do not immediately require as a reserve food supply for themselves or their seeds.

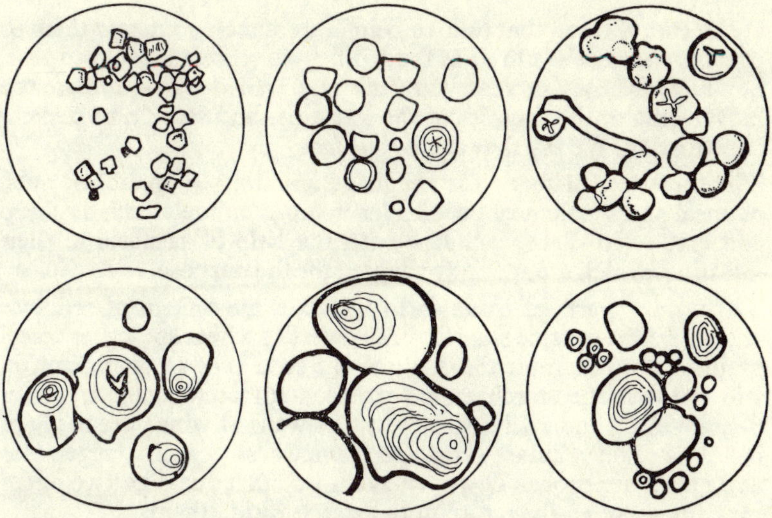

Starch grains, much magnified. Left to right:
top row—wheat, potato, sago bottom row—maize, tapioca, rice.

Some plants store starch in their stems, e.g., the sago palm; some in their tubers, e.g., the potato, and others in their roots, e.g., cassava from which tapioca is made. Starch is especially abundant in seeds, e.g., the cereals and pulses. Unripe fruits, such as apples and bananas, contain starch which changes into sugar as the fruits ripen. This insoluble stored-up starch in stems, tubers, roots and seeds can be readily converted back into soluble sugars when the plant requires. Some of our digestive juices are also able to bring about the same change.

When examined under a microscope starch is found to be in the form of minute cells or granules which vary in size and shape according to the plant from which they are derived. The starch is packed densely on the outside and before our digestive juices can change starch into glucose these "skins" must be broken open. This is done by cooking. Uncooked starchy foods such as raw potatoes, for example, are practically useless to us.

CELLULOSE

The term cellulose, used in a wide sense, covers a number of polysaccharides which are built up of thousands of sugar units. They are the most complicated of the carbohydrates. In fact, they are so complicated that human beings are unable to digest them so that they are useless to us as food. They do serve a useful purpose, however, for they increase the bulk of our food and stimulate the movements of the muscles of the intestines and so help to prevent constipation. We say they act as *roughage*.

The most useful foods for roughage are fruits, vegetables, nuts, oatmeal and wholemeal bread. Herbivorous animals such as sheep and cattle can digest cellulose with the help of bacteria in their intestines which are specially adapted for the purpose.

The stringy parts of fruits and vegetables are a form of cellulose and so are the outside skins or bran layers of wheat and other cereal grains. If you examine the diagram of a section of a raw potato you will see that the starch grains are each surrounded by a skin of denser starch and enclosed in cells, the walls of which are made of cellulose. The cellulose skins and frameworks of fruits, vegetables and grains are broken down by cooking so that our digestive juices may the more easily act upon the starch inside them.

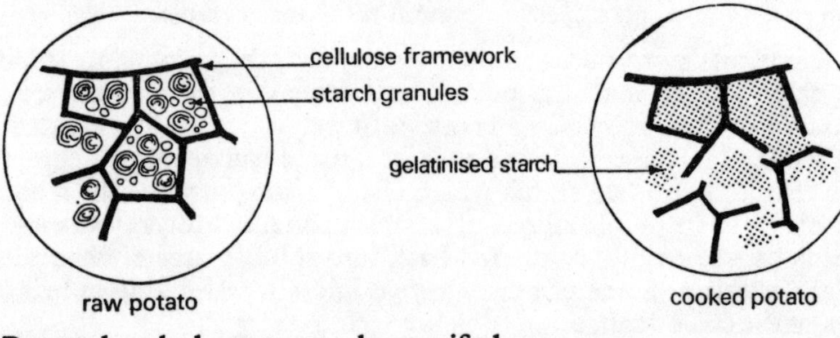

Raw and cooked potato, much magnified.

From the *Manual of Nutrition*, by permission of the Controller, H.M.S.O.

Pectin is another complicated carbohydrate. It is this substance which forms a jelly when fruit is made into jam. Without sufficient pectin fruit cannot be made to set into jam.

Dextrin is another complicated carbohydrate intermediate between starch and maltose. Dextrin is formed from starch by our digestive juices as an intermediate stage in its conversion to glucose. Starch is partly changed into dextrin when starchy foods are cooked as in crust of bread and toast.

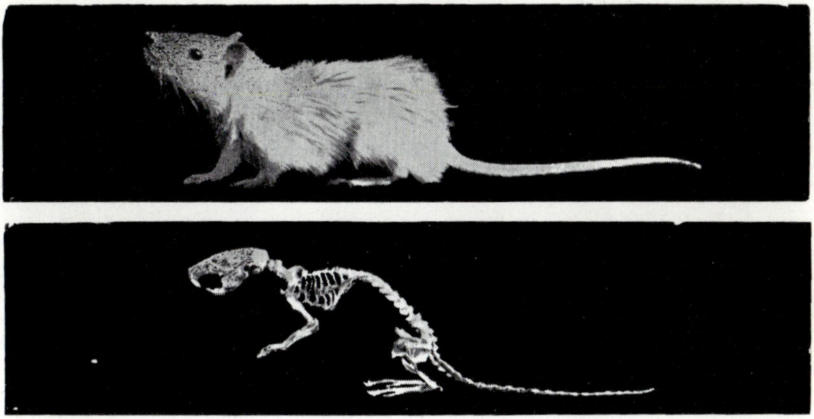

This rat ate only meat, potato, bread and butter. He weighed 89 grammes when 6 months old. His bones also show the effects of poor diet.

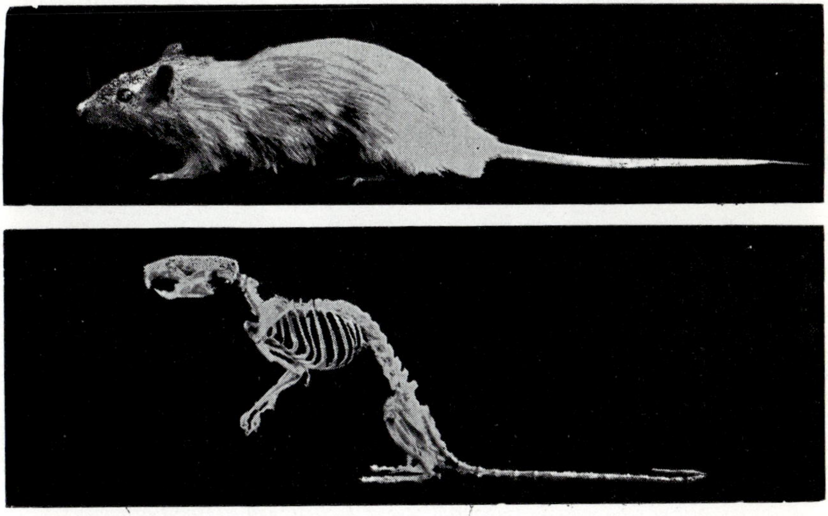

His twin brother ate plenty of milk and vegetables, besides meat, potato, bread and butter. He weighed 194 grammes at 6 months. His bones are strong and well formed.

By courtesy of US Bureau of Home Economics

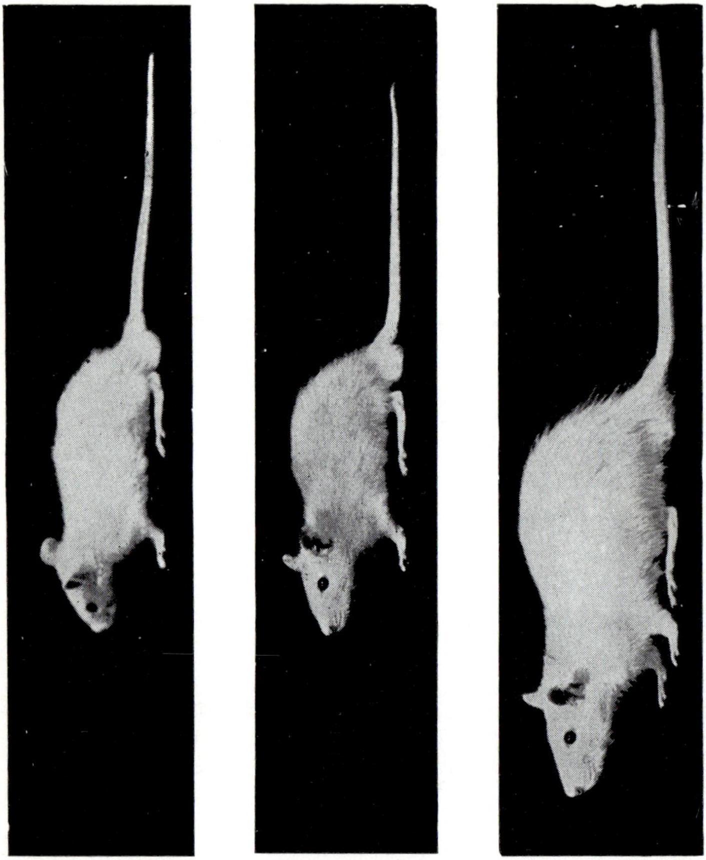

PROTEINS FOR BUILDING TISSUES

Rats from the same litter, 11 weeks old.

Left-hand rat had good protein, but not enough. It weighed 70 grammes.

Centre rat had enough protein, but of a poor kind. It weighed only 65 grammes.

Right-hand rat had good protein and plenty of it. It grew normally and weighed 193 grammes.

By courtesy of US Bureau of Home Economics

VITAMIN A

Rats from the same litter, 11 weeks old.

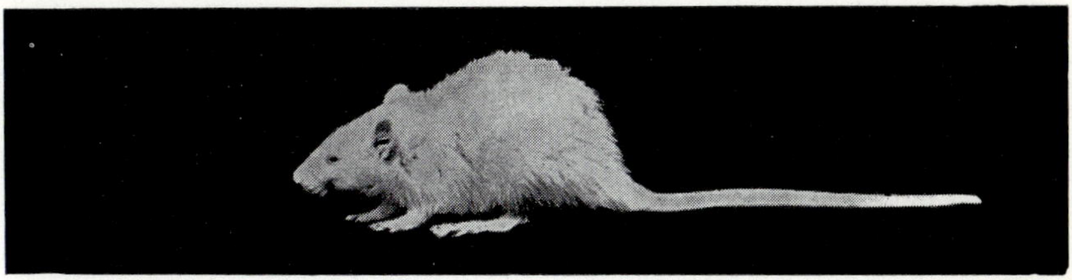

This rat had no Vitamin A. It weighed only 56 grammes and had infected eyes, rough fur and showed lack of vigour.

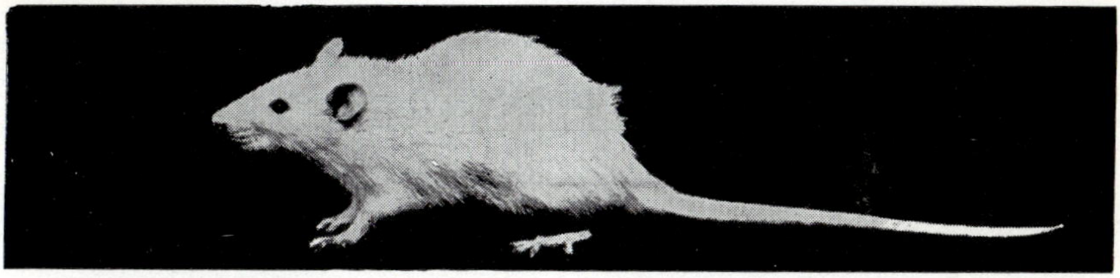

This rat had plenty of Vitamin A and weighed 123 grammes. It had bright eyes, sleek fur and was vigorous.

By courtesy of US Bureau of Home Economics

VITAMIN B_1

This rat did not have enough Vitamin B_1 and suffered from lack of muscle control (spastic paralysis).

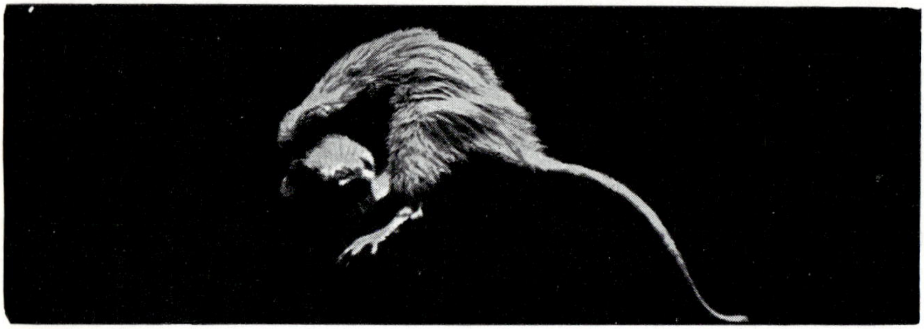

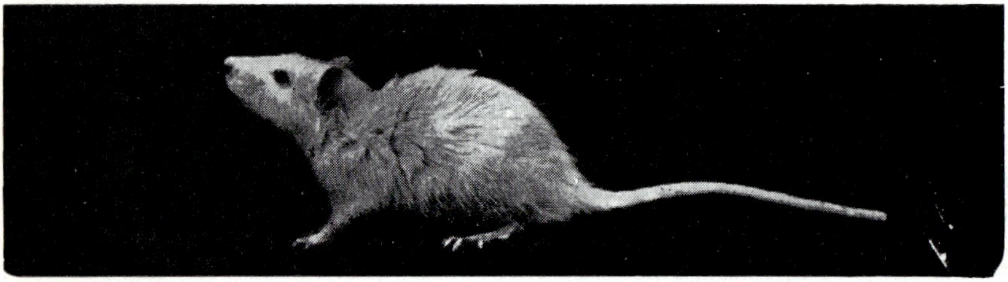

The same rat 24 hours later, after receiving a food rich in Vitamin B_1. It has then recovered muscle control.

By courtesy of US Bureau of Home Economics

VITAMIN C

Guinea pigs of the same age.

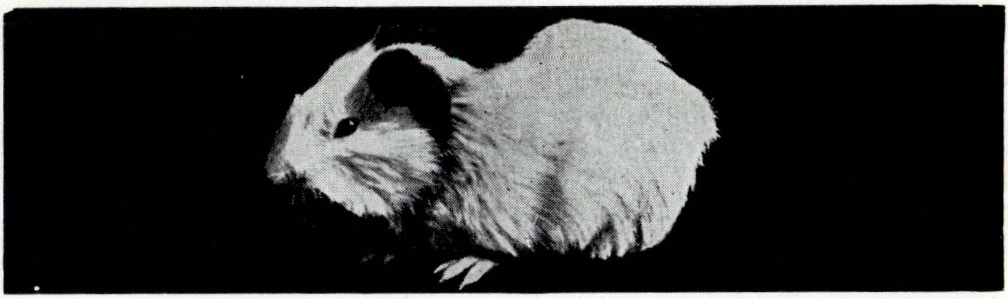

This had no Vitamin C and developed scurvy. Note its rough fur and crouched position due to sore joints.

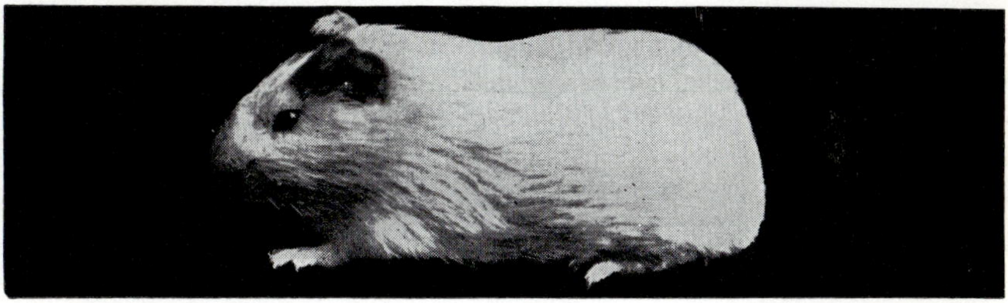

This had plenty of Vitamin C. It has sleek fur and is healthy and alert.

By courtesy of US Bureau of Home Economics

VITAMIN D

Rats from the same litter, 20 weeks old.

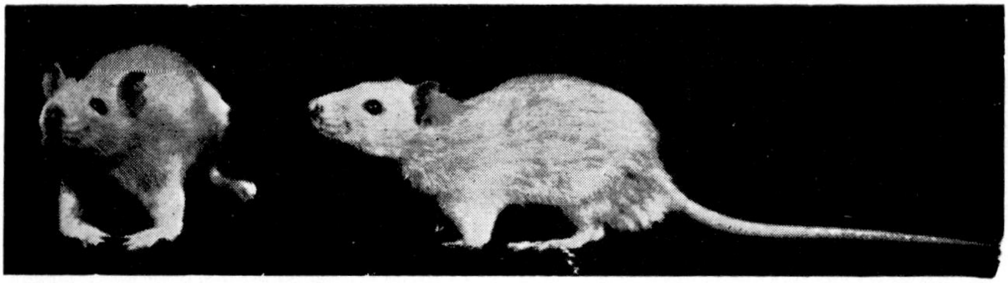

This rat had no Vitamin D and showed the short body and bow legs typical of rickets.

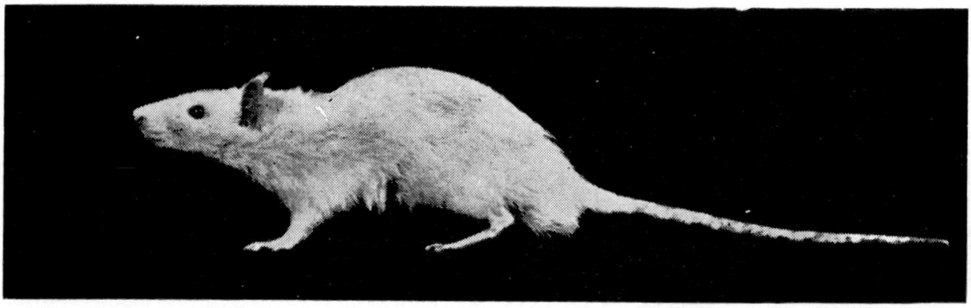

This rat had plenty of Vitamin D; its bones are strong and straight.

By courtesy of US Bureau of Home Economics

Rats from the same litter, 11 weeks old.

This rat lacked calcium. It weighed 91 grammes and showed the short stubby legs due to poorly formed bones.

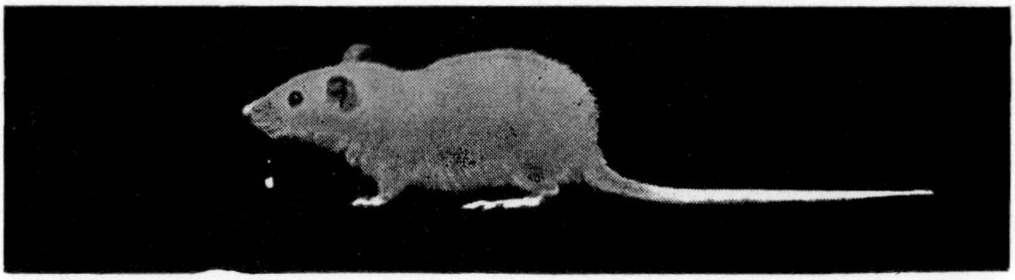

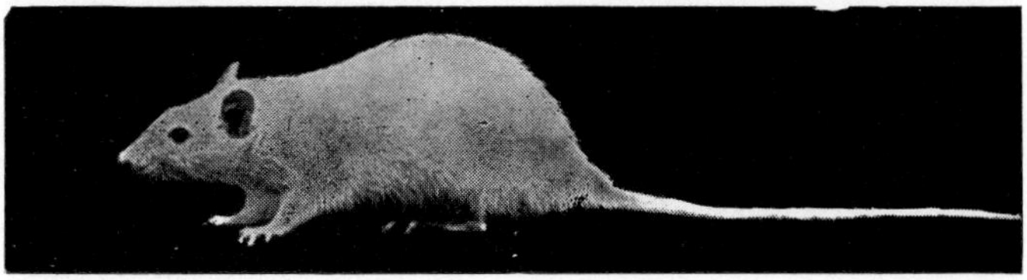

This rat had an abundance of calcium. It weighed 219 grammes and its bones were well formed.

Rats from the same litter, 9 weeks old.

This rat did not have enough phosphorus. It grew slowly and weighed only 60 grammes.

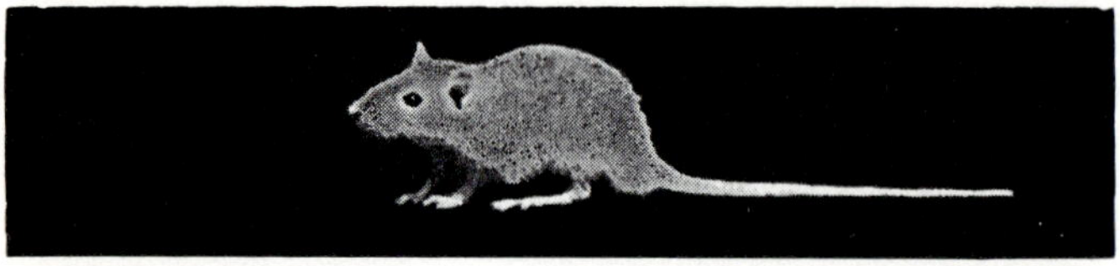

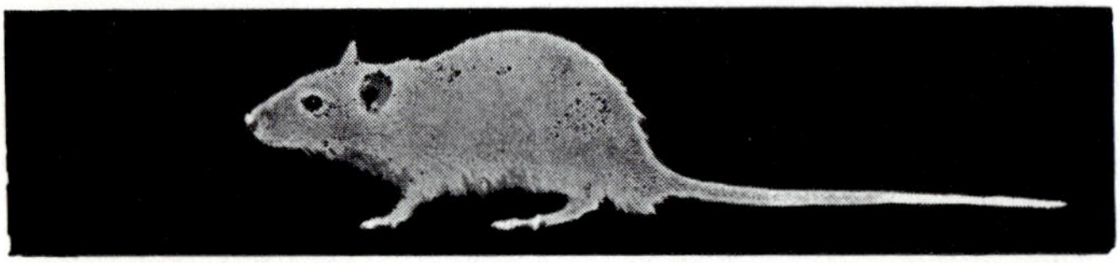

This rat had plenty of phosphorus and weighed 115 grammes.

By courtesy of US Bureau of Home Economics

Crust and toast are more digestible than ordinary bread. They need more chewing, are more intimately mixed with saliva, enter the stomach in smaller pieces and provide greater surface area for the digestive juices to work on.

We eat many more carbohydrate foods than any others and starch is our main carbohydrate. In most countries, cereals provide the bulk of the food starch. Wheat, largely in the form of bread, is the staple cereal in this country while rice is "the staff of life" in eastern countries, viz., China, Japan and India. Potatoes come a good second as sources of food starch in this country. Other foods besides wheat, rice and potatoes which consist largely of starch are sago, tapioca and arrowroot.

Besides being valuable energy foods, carbohydrates serve two other useful purposes in our diet. As previously stated, fat is a more concentrated energy food but our bodies have greater difficulty in completely burning fat than they have in burning carbohydrate. When carbohydrate and fat are eaten together, as in bread and butter, our bodies can burn the fat more completely just as a coal fire will burn better if we start it with paper and wood. Too much fat with too little carbohydrate might upset digestion.

Carbohydrates are also sometimes referred to as *protein sparers* because unless protein and carbohydrate are eaten together the valuable amino-acids of the protein which should be used as body-builders and repairers will be largely wasted by being burnt up

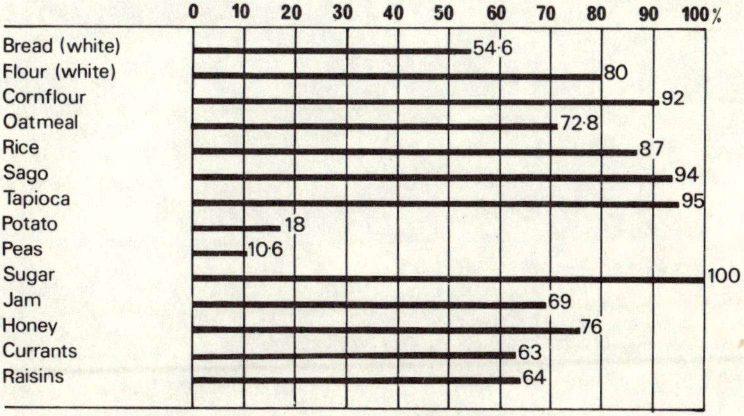

Percentages of carbohydrate in certain foods.

C

instead of carbohydrate to provide us with sufficient energy. Protein and carbohydrate should always be eaten together at the same meal. We do this, of course, when we eat fish and chips, meat and potatoes, and bread and cheese.

Because carbohydrate foods are plentiful, cheap, easily stored and readily prepared, there is a great danger that many people, particularly the poor, may eat too much of them and too little of the more expensive body-building and protective foods. Another danger when carbohydrate foods form too large a part of the diet is that some cereal foods, and particularly sugar, are very highly refined in the course of preparation and the protective materials, the minerals and vitamins, particularly thiamine, which they contain in their natural state, are removed. For this reason it is important not to eat too much of these highly refined foods and always to ensure that their deficiency in protective materials is made up for by eating other foods which contain useful amounts of minerals and vitamins, e.g., vegetables.

In any balanced diet, carbohydrates should provide the major part of our energy requirements. This means that more than half our energy should come from starchy and sugary foods.

Our main supplies of carbohydrates in the diet come from bread, sugar, flour, other cereals, potatoes and jam.

3 Fats

Like carbohydrates, i.e., starches and sugars, fats are made up of carbon, hydrogen and oxygen, but the proportion of oxygen is much less in fats than in carbohydrates. Since carbon and hydrogen are the substances which burn with oxygen, their greater proportion in fats explains why fats are more concentrated energy foods than carbohydrates. You will remember that the energy value of a fat is some 9 kcals per gramme compared with 4 kcals per gramme for average carbohydrates and proteins. Fats thus provide energy in a compact form.

Oils are the same as fats except that they are liquid instead of solid at ordinary temperatures. Oils can be solidified to fats by cooling and fats melted to oils by heating. The fats we eat are melted into oils by the heat of our stomachs. Some of the higher melting-point fats such as mutton fat (melting point 50° C) are not as quickly melted as lower melting-point fats such as butter (melting-point 32° C).

Fats and oils are found in both plants and animals and, in both cases, are formed from glucose by loss of oxygen and gain of energy. Chemically, fats and oils are composed of combinations of two kinds of simpler substances. One of them is the sweet sticky liquid known as *glycerin* or *glycerol* and the other is an acid. Because they are found in fats these acids are called *fatty acids*.

Among the twenty-five kinds of fatty acids found in food fats the commonest are palmitic acid, stearic acid and oleic acid. A less common one is butyric acid which is present in milk, cream and butter.

A fat is made by a combination of three molecules of fatty acid with one molecule of glycerol. The three fatty acids may be all the same or they may differ from each other. Thus palmitic and stearic acid may well both be present in the same fat.

The fatty acids may be saturated, or unsaturated. Saturated fatty acids contain their full complement of hydrogen atoms, they are relatively unreactive (e.g. they do not go rancid so quickly as the unsaturated fatty acids) and they form solid fats when combined with glycerol.

Saturated fatty acids include:— palmitic and stearic acids found in beef and mutton fat, butyric acid found in butter and caprylic acid found in coconut oil, and butter made from goat's or cow's milk.

Unsaturated fatty acids contain less than their full complement of hydrogen atoms, the double bond links that are present make the molecule reactive and it will easily be oxidised (i.e. go rancid). It is, however, also possible to insert extra hydrogen atoms into the molecule and thus convert it to a saturated fatty acid. This process is called hydrogenation; it will stabilise the molecule and incidentally convert the fat from liquid to solid.

Unsaturated fatty acids include:—oleic acid found in olive oil and in lard, linoleic acid found in corn oil, soya bean oil and linseed oil, and arachidonic acid found in some animal fats.

Some unsaturated fatty acids have more than one double bond. Three of these polyunsaturated fatty acids, linoleic, linolenic and arachidonic, are essential for children and adults. There is some evidence that unsaturated fats may help to reduce the risk of developing coronary heart disease.

The differences between natural food fats depend largely upon the proportions of palmitin, stearin and olein they contain. Beef and mutton fats contain large proportions of palmitin and stearin and so are hard fats. Lard contains a larger proportion of olein and so is a soft fat. Olive oil contains practically nothing but olein and, in consequence, is a liquid. Corn oil and groundnut oil are rich in polyunsaturated fatty acids.

Rancidity in fats is usually due to the oxidation of unsaturated fatty acids by the oxygen of the air and, to a lesser extent, to the action of micro-organisms and moulds. Anti-oxidants may be added to manufactured fats to prevent the fat from going rancid so easily.

Fats and oils are insoluble in water but, when treated with alkali, e.g., caustic soda, they form glycerol and soap, both of which are soluble. The process is called *saponification.* Only fats and oils which can be saponified can be used by the body as foods and sources of energy. Mineral oils, which have a totally different chemical structure, cannot be saponified. Mineral oils are not fats and are *not* a food.

The fat in our diet is supplied mainly by butter, cream, margarine, cooking oils, cheese, suet, dripping, the so-called fat fish such as herrings, salmon and sardines, and nuts such as Brazil nuts, peanuts, almonds and coconuts. The common vegetables contain practically no fat at all. The amount of fat in wheat flour and other cereal products is very small except in the case of oatmeal. Margarine is manufactured from a variety of fats and oils such as beef fat, lard, olive oil, peanut oil, soya bean oil, cotton seed oil and others, as well as specially treated fish oils.

Certain natural animal fats in this list are superior to the vegetable fats and oils in one important respect. In addition to being quite as good as vegetable fats and oils for energy purposes, the fats of butter, fat fish and liver contain protective material in the form of vitamins A and D which are not found in vegetable fats and oils. Margarine now has these vitamins added to it during the process of manufacture to make it equivalent to butter in protective value as well as energy value.

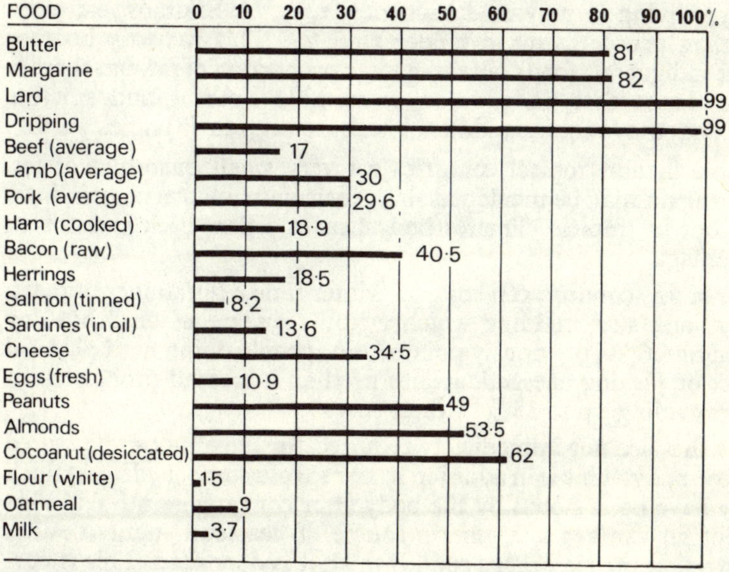

Percentages of fat in certain foods.

There does not appear to be any essential minimum amount of fat which must be eaten daily to maintain the body in good health. In this country the usual quantities of fat in the diets of adults provides something like 25% of their energy requirements. An average adult in this country consumes about 340 g. of fat weekly in the form of butter, margarine, lard, cooking fats and oils. With the fat, "visible" and "invisible", present in many other foods, a daily intake of about 85 g. is usual.

Since fat is such a concentrated energy food its use allows us to obtain our energy needs without overloading our stomachs. The less fat we eat the more carbohydrate we require and this is very bulky compared with fat. This is why children, who have small stomachs but big energy requirements, need a relatively large amount of easily digested fat.

Without fats for cooking and baking our food would be much less appetising and extremely monotonous. Fats are the most slowly digested of all our foods and, for this reason, meals containing fat are the most satisfying and the most lasting, and the lubricating action of fat makes meals easier to eat.

People living in very cold countries, e.g., the Eskimos, eat more fat than people living in milder climates. This is partly because their indigenous food contains a large proportion of fat, but there is little doubt that, in addition to suitable clothing and suitable housing, they require additional kcals. to keep their bodies warm.

People in hot tropical countries eat very small quantities of fat. This again may be incidental since their native foods contain little fat, but in tropical climates body heat is a drawback and not an advantage.

We, in this country, can enjoy in winter time a hot dinner of meat, gravy and suet pudding which would nauseate us on a hot day in summer. As previously pointed out, people doing hard physical work or playing energetic games need an increased proportion of fat providing up to 35% of their energy.

Fats that are not immediately required for burning can be stored by the body. This is in addition to any surplus carbohydrates which may have been stored by the body after conversion into fat. This depot fat can act as a reserve source of heat and energy besides protecting certain organs round which it is deposited. This is particularly true of the kidneys which are quickly affected by cold. The layer of fat round the kidneys has an insulating action and keeps them warm. Thin people feel the cold more quickly than the plump who have the advantage of an insulating layer of fat just under the skin.

It is worth while pointing out again that fat foods should always be eaten along with carbohydrate foods as we ordinarily do in a normal mixed diet. Otherwise the fats will be incompletely burnt to form substances which cause headaches and sickness, and loss of appetite. Examples of carbohydrate and fat eaten together include such things as bread and butter, strawberries and cream, cakes, pastry, suet pudding and chips. Perhaps you can think of other examples.

EMULSIFIERS

These are substances that may be added to fats during their manufacture. They will help the fat to disperse and thus make it easier to mix or they can make the fat easier to spread, or can help to prevent spluttering. There are a considerable number of emulsifiers. Their use is controlled by law.

4 Proteins

The word protein is derived from a Greek word meaning "I am first," and in all living things proteins are of first importance. As pointed out in Chapter 1, proteins are essential because the cells of all forms of life, whether animal or vegetable, are built up of the jelly-like material called *protoplasm* which consists of protein. There can be no life without proteins; they are the very basis of life.

Like carbohydrates and fats, proteins contain carbon, hydrogen and oxygen, but, in addition, they always contain *nitrogen.* Some proteins also contain sulphur and some few contain phosphorus. Proteins are far more complicated substances than either carbohydrates or fats. They are, in fact, the most complicated substances known to science.

Plants can build up their proteins for themselves from the carbon dioxide they obtain from air, and from the water and mineral substances containing nitrogen (nitrates) which they obtain from soil. A few plants, known as *legumes,* such as peas, beans and clover, with the help of bacteria in nodules on their roots, can make use of the nitrogen in air to build up their proteins. Animals and human beings are unable to make proteins from either the nitrates of the soil or the nitrogen of the air. They depend completely upon proteins already made in plants or other animals. Thus proteins have all come from plants. "All flesh is grass."

There are thousands of different plant proteins and thousands of different animal and human proteins. And plant, animal, and human proteins, are all different from one another. Our particular proteins naturally very closely resemble animal proteins. All the myriad proteins, however, are alike in one respect. They are all built up of simpler substances known as *amino-acids* of which about twenty different ones may be present in a protein. They are linked together, often in thousands, in chains folded in upon themselves.

Proteins differ from one another in the number, the kind and the arrangement of the amino-acids they contain. A particular amino-acid may be present in large amount in one protein, present in very small amount in a second protein and completely absent in a third. There are at least twenty-two different kinds of amino-acids found in proteins. Imagine a large number of each of twenty-two differently coloured kinds of beads. They would make an enormous number of strings of beads all different from one another. They would differ in almost every conceivable way—in either the total number of beads, or the numbers of different kinds of beads or in the order in which we grouped them on the string. Now, perhaps, you will appreciate why proteins are such complicated substances.

Below are given diagrams which may help you still further. We will take only twelve beads and suppose there are three each of four different kinds shown by different letters of the alphabet like this.

A, A, A.	B, B, B.	C, C, C.	D, D, D.
1st kind of bead	2nd kind of bead	3rd kind of bead	4th kind of bead

Then we might arrange some of them in a set like this:
No. I. —A—A—A—B—B—B—D—D—

or like this:
No. II. —A—A—C—C—D—B—B—A—D—B—C—D—

You will see that Set No. I differs from Set No. II because:
(1) It has a different total number of beads.
(2) It has different numbers of the different kinds of beads.
(3) The beads are differently arranged.
(4) One kind of bead (—C—) is completely absent.

It is in ways such as these that the twenty-two different amino-acids can join together to form different proteins in vast numbers.

When we digest protein foods our digestive juices break up the proteins into their different amino-acids. As these amino-acids are circulated in our blood, each cell of the body chooses for its growth and repair the amounts and the kinds of amino-acids it requires. Any surplus amino-acids which are not required at the time for growth and repair are burnt as fuel to supply heat and energy. The kcal. value in the body of proteins is much the same as that of carbohydrates, i.e., about 4 kcal/g.

The body is able to change some amino-acids it does not need into amino-acids that it does need. There are, however, eight amino-acids needed by adults, with one, or possibly two, additional ones needed by growing children which cannot be made by the body and must, therefore, be supplied in the diet. These are called the *essential amino-acids*. Without these essential amino-acids the growth and repair of body tissues are impossible.

Proteins which contain these essential amino-acids in satisfactory proportions will obviously be better body builders and repairers and, consequently, more valuable foods than proteins from which one or more of the essential amino-acids is missing. Such proteins are said to have a high biological value. Generally speaking, the animal proteins such as those in milk, cheese, eggs, meat and fish contain all the essential amino-acids and have high biological value. Plant proteins, such as those in cereals, pulses and nuts, generally have one or more of the essential amino-acids either missing or in short supply. They have, therefore, a lower biological value than animal proteins, but are useful in a supplementary capacity.

There are, however, some exceptions to this rule, e.g., soya beans and gelatine. Soya bean flour contains the essential amino-acids although it is a plant product. Soya beans have been used for centuries by the Chinese and Japanese as their main source of protein. Gelatine is an animal protein made by boiling bones and gristle. It is used in making table jellies and it is gelatine which causes meat stock to set to a jelly. Gelatine lacks one of the essential amino-acids and so has a low biological value.

The fact that the proteins of gelatine and the plant proteins of bread, flour, oatmeal, peas, beans, lentils and nuts have essential amino-acids missing does not mean that they are not valuable to us. They are, and we can best make use of them by taking them as supplementary body-builders. In fact, by mixing them with animal proteins we get the best out of both animal and plant proteins.

Returning to the simile of the beads, if we assume that the ideal protein for us to eat (that with a biological value of 100%) contains beads ABCD in the proportions of 10A:9B:8C:7D, a high biological value protein might then well contain beads 20A:10B:8C:7D. In other words too many A and B beads. A lower biological value protein might well contain only 8B:8C:7D; if now you were to eat these two proteins together it can be seen that the excess A and B beads in the one protein will make up the deficiency in the other so that together these two proteins have an ideal biological value.

In terms of real foods meat and peas eaten together at the same meal will supply us with more body-building material than if they were eaten at separate meals. Any amino-acids which may be present in small amounts or completely missing from one protein food can be made up from another protein food in which they are present in large amounts. The more varied the body-building foods we eat, the more likely we are to supply our bodies with the amounts and the kinds of amino-acids they need.

Gelatine is rich in the essential amino-acid, lysine, in which cereal proteins are deficient. Thus, when beef tea and toast are eaten together the gelatine provides the amino-acids lacking in the toast and the combination improves the nutritive value of each. A similar enhancement of total protein value is achieved in a meal combining eggs, cheese or milk with bread.

It is usually reckoned that the best results are achieved if we obtain half our protein from animal foods and half from plant foods. Remember, too, that proteins will be less likely to be wasted as fuel if eaten along with carbohydrate food. We shall make the best use of our protein foods and obtain their maximum value if we eat them along with carbohydrate in small amounts at each meal rather than eating a large amount at one meal, say dinner, and practically none at other meals of the day. Unfortunately, amino-acids, unlike carbohydrates and fats, cannot be stored in the body.

A further factor in the assessment of protein values of foods must be that of their digestibility. Some protein foods (e.g. cheese) are difficult to digest and so amino-acids cannot be fully absorbed. The digestibility of the food × biological value is known as the *net protein utilisation value* (N.P.U.) and is highest for human milk and eggs.

Protein foods are the most expensive foods. This is particularly true in the case of animal proteins. They are also the most tasty and appetising and give a feeling of being well-fed which carbohydrates never do. There is consequently a danger that the father of the family may, in some instances, get more than his share of meat, fish and eggs, and the mother and children less than they ought. Their need for protein foods may well be as much as his. Growing children, and young persons generally, need a good share of animal proteins, such as those of meat, fish and dairy products—milk, cheese and eggs. They can scarcely have too much milk.

Children should not, as sometimes happens, be given gravy only with potatoes while the grown-ups get meat and potatoes, or chips only while the adults have fish and chips.

The table below gives recommended protein requirements.

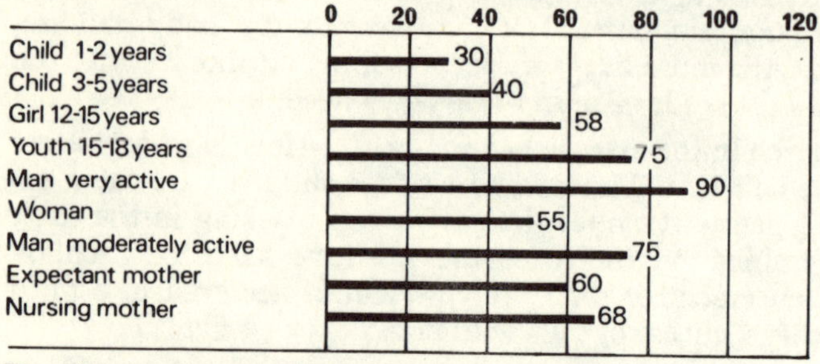

Protein requirements in grammes per day.

Our main supplies of protein in the diet come from meat, dairy produce, bread, flour and other cereals.

It is now considered that adults are receiving a satisfactory supply of protein if 11% of their total kcals. intake is derived from protein. Children and adolescents who are still growing, expectant and

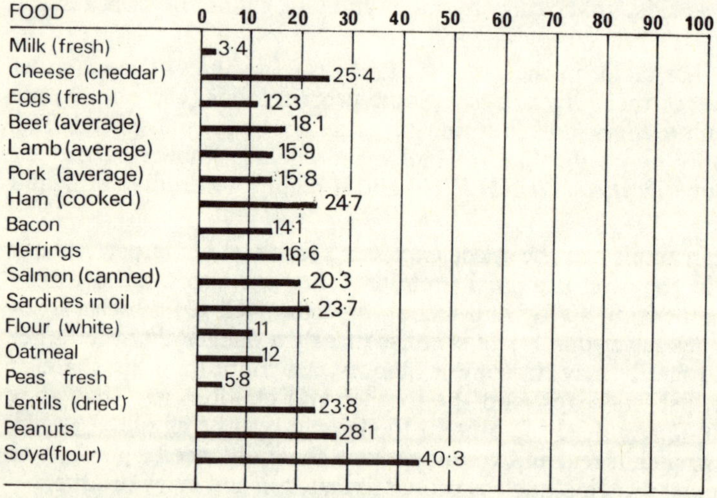

Percentages of proteins in certain foods.

nursing mothers, should have sufficient protein to provide 14% of their total kcals.

In some parts of the world there is a great deficiency of protein in the diet and this is particularly noticeable in the children, whose growth is stunted. Gross deficiency shows in the typical starvation symptoms of distended stomach and matchstick limbs, a condition known as Kwashiorkor.

5 Minerals and Water

We have seen that carbohydrates and fats consist of carbon, hydrogen and oxygen, and that proteins, in addition to these three elements, always contain nitrogen and sometimes sulphur and phosphorus. The term *minerals* is applied to elements other than carbon, hydrogen, oxygen and nitrogen which are found in the body and which must be provided in our food.

"Minerals" is not a particularly good name for them because they are not minerals in the sense that limestone and iron ore are minerals, nor are they minerals in the sense that lemonade is a mineral. Yet they are minerals in the sense that they form the ash left behind when bodies are cremated and the dust left behind when bodies decay underground. All have been derived originally from the soil and ultimately return to it.

This ash has been analysed and found to contain the surprisingly large number of nineteen different mineral elements. Their total weight amounts to about one-twentieth of the weight of the body.

Some of them are present in very large proportions while others are present in such minute quantities that their amounts are described as being "traces" or even "mere traces." Yet even these "traces" and "mere traces" have been proved essential to health. Each and every one of them is necessary and no one mineral can do the work of another. Each of them must be supplied in our food.

The mineral substances present in largest amounts are calcium and phosphorus. In the form of calcium phosphate (phosphate of lime) they form the principal constituents of bones and teeth which account for a very large proportion of the weight of minerals in the body. Potassium, sulphur, chlorine, sodium, magnesium, iron, manganese and iodine are present in much smaller amounts while the remaining nine minerals—silicon, cobalt, boron, arsenic, fluorine, copper, zinc, aluminium and nickel—are present as traces or mere traces.

The minerals are used by the body for three main purposes:

(1) They build up the bones and teeth.
(2) They are essential constituents of every cell in the body. Muscle cells, nerve cells, liver cells, brain cells and so on, all contain minerals.
(3) All the fluids which circulate in the body, such as the blood, the lymph, the digestive juices and so on, contain minerals. For example: blood, sweat, and tears, taste of salt.

Many of the minerals are needed in such small quantities and are present in so many different foods that there is little likelihood of our not getting sufficient of them. Others are either needed in much larger quantities or are not present in all foods and consequently there is a danger of a shortage of them in our bodies. Among these are calcium, iron, iodine and fluorine, and, from our point of view, these four minerals require special notice.

Minerals are continually being lost from the body through:

(1) The kidneys, in the urine.
(2) The skin, in perspiration.
(3) The bowels, in faeces.

These lost minerals must be replaced or health will suffer. In the case of growing children the minerals taken into the body must more than replace those lost, otherwise normal growth such as the formation of bone and building up of tissue will be impossible.

Foods vary greatly in the amounts of each mineral which they contain. A particular food may be a good source of one mineral and a poor source of another. Milk, for instance, is particularly rich in calcium and phosphorus but poor in iron.

Unfortunately, too, the body is not always able to make full use of the minerals which may be present in a particular food. This is especially true of calcium, phosphorus and iron as will be explained later. Though present in a food they are not always *available* to the body.

All foods in their natural state contain some minerals but the amounts are always much less than those of carbohydrates, fats and proteins. In fact, it is exceptional to find a natural food which contains as much as 1% of a particular mineral. Many of the refining and milling processes to which some foods are subjected reduce the amounts still further.

CALCIUM AND PHOSPHORUS

Calcium is the mineral which is present in the body in the largest amount. It is mainly required to form the calcium phosphate of which our bones and teeth are largely composed. In addition, calcium is necessary for the normal working of our muscles and the proper growth of children. Blood will not clot during bleeding unless it contains a certain definite proportion of calcium. This proportion is controlled by the parathyroid glands (small glands attached to the thyroid gland in the neck); calcium is withdrawn from the bones, if necessary, or deposited in the bones if there is too much in the blood.

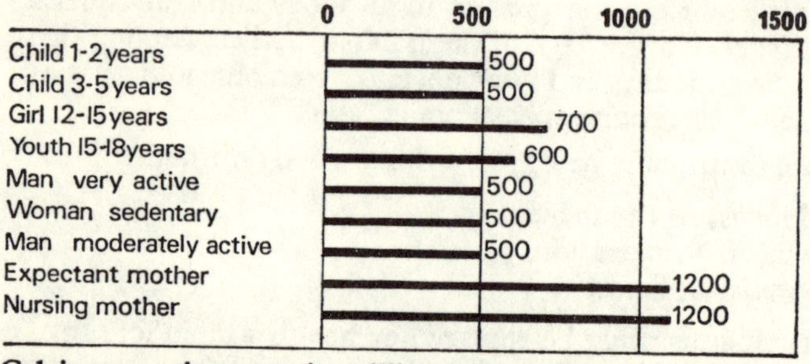

Calcium requirements in milligrammes per day.

Phosphorus is the mineral in the body which comes next to calcium in amount. It is used mainly in the formation of bones and teeth but is also found in all the tissues of the body and in every cell of the body, being an ingredient of some of the most important proteins. It plays an important part in the release of energy from food.

When a baby is born its bones are soft and pliable because they consist largely of cartilage or gristle. To convert this gristle into hard, solid bone, calcium and phosphorus must be deposited in it. As will be explained in the chapter on vitamins, vitamin D is also necessary for this process to take place. Should any of these three things—calcium, phosphorus and vitamin D—be lacking, bones and teeth will not form properly and rickets and decayed teeth may result.

Phosphorus is much more common in foods than is calcium. There is little likelihood of our getting too little phosphorus, even though the body cannot always utilise all the phosphorus in food, but there is a danger of getting too little calcium. The danger is greatest in the cases of infants, growing children and expectant and nursing mothers, who need increased amounts of calcium. A growing child needs, in proportion to its size, about twice as much calcium as an adult. The need for calcium in old age is sometimes overlooked; insufficient may help to cause the brittle bones of old age.

There are only a few foods which contain really substantial amounts of calcium. Our main sources of calcium in the diet are milk, milk powder, cheese, bread, flour and green vegetables. Milk is the finest of all foods for building bones and teeth.

When we eat the bones of fish, as we do with whitebait, sprats, sardines and tinned salmon, they supply us with valuable calcium. "Hard" water also contains calcium salts which help to supplement our supplies of food calcium. During and since World War II calcium carbonate (creta praeparata) has been added to all flours, except true wholemeal flour, at the rate of 1 lb to 320 lb sack to help to overcome the danger of calcium shortage in the diet. Eggs, turnip, oatmeal and nuts are other foods which contain useful amounts of calcium.

Unfortunately, our bodies are not always able to make full use of all the calcium in foods. Some of it may be in an insoluble form which cannot pass through the walls of the intestines into the blood stream. In the bran of cereal grains, such as wheat and oats, is a substance called *phytic acid* which may combine with the calcium in other foods to form an insoluble calcium compound and thus make the calcium *unavailable*. Fortunately, during breadmaking with yeast much of the phytic acid in the flour is destroyed by the yeast so that little of its calcium is lost to the body. *Oxalic acid* is another acid which can form an insoluble compound with calcium. Oxalic acid is found in rhubarb and spinach, but we normally eat so little of these foods that their effect can be ignored.

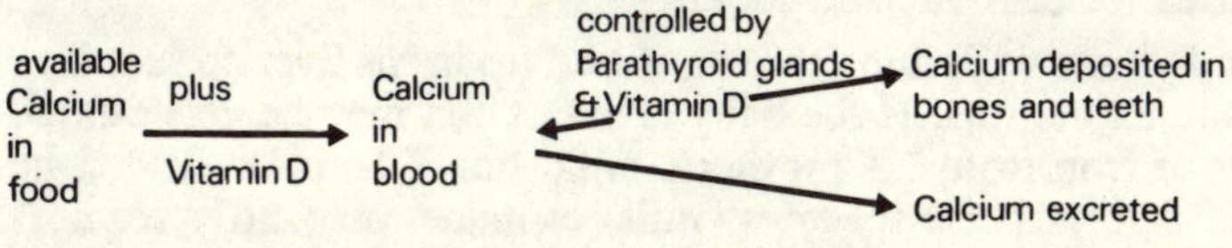

IRON

Iron is present in the *haemoglobin* of the red corpuscles of the blood which absorb oxygen from the air we breathe into our lungs. Lack

D

of iron leads to lack of haemoglobin which, in its turn, leads to lack of oxygen for burning up our fuel foods to provide energy. This explains the listlessness characteristic of *anaemia*, which is sometimes described as "the occupational disease" of the British housewife.

The body takes great care to preserve as much of its iron as possible. When red corpuscles become worn out, as they are continually doing, they are broken up in the liver, but the liver retains the iron of the old red corpuscles to use in making new ones. This building up of new red corpuscles takes place in a rather unexpected place—the marrow of the bones.

Nevertheless there is always a small loss of iron in the various secretions and in the general wear and tear of the body. Larger losses occur during bleeding and, in the case of women and girls, during menstruation and pregnancy. These losses must be made good by the provision of iron in their food.

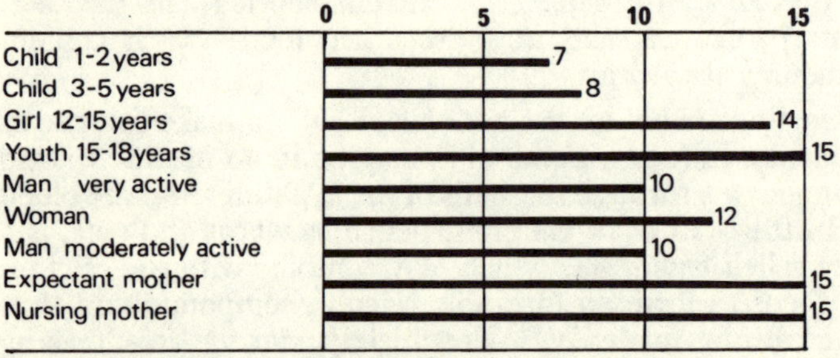

Iron requirements in milligrammes per day.

The best foods for supplying iron are liver and kidneys, meat, egg yolk, almonds, raisins, bread, flour, potatoes and cabbage, and useful amounts of iron may be supplied to the body from the water used for drinking and cooking.

A baby is born with enough iron stored up in his liver to last him for about six months. If the baby is breast-fed then he gets a small amount of iron from his mother's milk, but if he is bottle-fed he gets much less because cows' milk contains very little iron. A bottle-fed baby is thus liable to become anaemic after the age of six months. However, nowadays it is normal for all babies to be on to mixed feeds before this age and iron will be present in those containing egg, meat, green vegetables and fortified cereals.

The absorption of iron from the food is apparently very difficult, and the factors influencing it are not yet fully understood. It seems, however, that in order to appreciably increase the quantity of iron absorbed very large doses have to be given, and Vitamin C is thought to help in the absorption of iron.

As in the case of calcium and phosphorus, the iron in foods is not always available to the body because it may be in an insoluble form. Phytic acid and oxalic acid, which can combine with calcium to make it unavailable to the body, can do the same with iron. Spinach is an example of a food which contains iron in an insoluble form which is thus useless to the body. It is very doubtful if most of the iron in "red" meat, liver and "black puddings" is available to the body.

IODINE

Iodine has already been mentioned as an essential substance for the thyroid glands in the neck. The secretion of the thyroid glands, *thyroxine*, consists largely of iodine which must be supplied in the food if these important glands are to work efficiently.

Without an adequate amount of iodine, the thyroid glands cannot secrete sufficient thyroxine and a form of *goitre* is likely to result. In extreme cases, the children of mothers suffering from goitre are born with inactive thyroid glands. Since the thyroid glands control physical and mental growth, such children become deformed idiots or *cretins*, but, in some cases, can be made normal by being fed with preparations of animal thyroid glands.

Iodine is derived mainly from sea foods—sea fish, oysters, mussels, and so on. In addition, water used for drinking and cooking sometimes contains iodine and so do vegetables, particularly watercress and onions, which have been grown in soil containing traces of iodine.

In spite of the very small amount of iodine needed by the body there are parts of the world where insufficient is present in food and drinking water. These districts are usually far removed from the sea or are mountainous, particularly limestone districts. Sea water contains iodine which is carried in sea spray several miles inland by the wind and thus finds its way into soil and drinking water and into the vegetables grown in such soil.

In some parts of America, in Switzerland and, in this country, in the hilly districts of Derbyshire, Yorkshire, Cumberland and

Gloucestershire there is insufficient iodine in the soil and drinking water and, consequently, in the local vegetables. Goitre is relatively common in these districts. In this country, goitre is often referred to as "Derbyshire neck."

Where such lack of iodine occurs it is wise practice to use salt with small amounts of iodine compounds (iodised salt) for cooking and at the table. Natural unrefined salt contains iodine compounds but these are removed during the process of refining. Iodised sweets and chocolate have also been recommended for children living in such districts. The improvement in communications resulting in transport of fresh vegetables and other foods and the increased use of canned and frozen foods has helped to minimise these local deficiencies.

FLUORINE

Is a constituent of bones and teeth, but very little is found in foods, except fish and tea. Fluorine, however, occurs naturally in almost all water supplies, but in varying amounts. Where drinking water is deficient in fluorine, dental decay, especially among children, is much more prevalent. By the addition of sodium fluoride to drinking water so as to bring the concentration of fluorine to one part per million the deplorable state of children's teeth in this country would be enormously improved. Excessive amounts of fluorine can cause teeth to mottle with chalky white particles but the likelihood of that happening in this country is extremely remote.

The other mineral elements are present in so many foods that there is little risk of our not getting sufficient of them.

The following table shows the foods which contain the three minerals calcium, iron and iodine. These are to us the important ones because they are the ones most likely to be deficient in the diet.

Mineral	*Main sources in the diet*
Calcium	Milk, cheese, bread, flour, green vegetables.
Iron	Bread, flour, cereals, meat, potatoes, green vegetables, eggs.
Iodine	Sea fish, oysters, mussels. Vegetables, e.g., watercress, onions. Water. Iodised salt.

The chief sources of the essential mineral constituents of the diet are milk, cheese, eggs, green vegetables, potatoes, bread and fish.

The same fact will be noticeable when we study the vitamins. Consequently these are amongst the most valuable of our foods.

SALT (SODIUM CHLORIDE)

Common salt is a compound of sodium and chlorine, known as sodium chloride. It is present in all the fluids of the body in a definite amount and it is essential that this amount should always be accurately maintained.

A shortage of salt is likely to result in cramp of the muscles, but so many of our foods contain large amounts of salt, and we use so much salt for seasoning and flavouring our food, that there is little probability of our being short of it.

Salt is lost from the body in the urine and in perspiration. For this reason, we may need additional salt during hot weather or after violent exercise. Stokers, steel workers and miners, who work in hot places, and people who live in hot countries, require additional salt to make up for the large amount lost in heavy perspiration. Troops campaigning in the tropical forests of Burma experienced cramps which were relieved by salt.

The chlorine of salt is used by the body to form the hydrochloric acid of the gastric juice of the stomach which helps in the digestion of proteins.

Salt in excess of the body's needs is removed by the kidneys in the urine. For good health it is essential to maintain a balance between the salt and water intakes.

Foods which contain appreciable amounts of salt include cheese, kippers, ham, bacon, bread, butter and margarine.

WATER

Water is not commonly regarded as a food in the ordinary sense of the word but it is, nevertheless, of the very greatest importance in the diet. It is possible to live for several weeks without solid food but we can survive for a few days only without water. The body's need for water is indicated by thirst just as the need for food is indicated by hunger.

Nearly three-quarters of the weight of the body is made up of water. Every tissue and organ in the body—even bone—contains water. All the processes which take place in the body do so in a watery medium. Water is essential for the digestion and absorption of all our foods and for their transport throughout the body. Water is the great purifying agent in the body and removes waste materials in perspiration, urine and faeces. We can thus realise the important role played by water in building our bodies and safeguarding our health.

Water is continually being lost from the body through the skin, the lungs, the kidneys and the bowels. The body obtains its water mainly from the fluids we drink. These include, in addition to water itself, such beverages as tea, coffee, cocoa, milk, lemonade, and so on.

Secondly, the body obtains water from the solid foods we eat. Many solid foods contain surprisingly large amounts of water. Fresh fruit, for example, may contain from 70 to over 90% of water. Potatoes contain about 80% of water and turnips about 90%. Even a "dry" food such as white bread contains 39% of water while foods such as dried peas, lentils, milk powder, and dried egg still contain up to as much as 15% of water.

Finally, the body obtains water from the oxidation of energy foods. Fats and carbohydrates are ultimately oxidised in the body to carbon dioxide and water. The carbon they contain is oxidised to carbon dioxide (CO_2) and the hydrogen to water (H_2O).

The following table gives the approximate amounts of water which are usually reckoned as being taken in and lost by the body each day. Under normal conditions these amounts balance each other. Any necessary adjustment is made by the kidneys which excrete a larger, or a smaller, amount of urine.

Water taken in	
As drink	1·4 litres
In food	0·85 „
Formed in the body by oxidation of food	0·15 „
	2·4 litres

Water given out	
In urine	1·65 litres
From skin	0·6 ,,
From lungs	0·11 ,,
In faeces	0·04 ,,
	2·4 litres

These are, of course, average figures which will vary for obvious reasons, particularly the amount of perspiration. Nevertheless, they serve a useful purpose in showing that many people drink far too little water.

It is sometimes said that we should not drink much fluid with meals because this will dilute the digestive juices and weaken digestion. For a normal healthy person this is not true. The important thing is not when we drink but how much we drink.

6 Vitamins

The most important advance in our knowledge of foods made during this century has been the discovery of a number of previously unknown nutrients which are absolutely essential to health and, indeed, to life itself. Up to the beginning of the century it was thought that a diet which provided carbohydrate, fat, protein, minerals and water in suitable amounts was all that was necessary for maintaining health and activity. The Cambridge scientist Dr. (later Sir) Frederick Gowland Hopkins carried out a long series of experiments on the feeding of rats. He fed a group of them on carefully purified carbohydrates, fats, proteins, minerals and water. They failed to grow, soon began to lose weight and generally showed many signs of ill-health. Other rats were also fed on this purified diet but with the addition of a few drops of fresh milk, yeast extract or swede juice at different times of the day. These rats remained fit and active and grew at a normal rate. The rats which had been losing weight on the purified diet were then given a little milk in addition and, at once, they began to increase in weight and to become healthy again. The rats which had originally been given milk were now given the purified diet only. They soon stopped growing and began to lose weight.

In 1912 Hopkins published the results of his experiments and suggested that in natural foods there are a number of substances additional to carbohydrates, fats, proteins and minerals which are no less essential ingredients of a complete diet. He called them *accessory food factors*.

At about the same time, two pairs of American scientists, Osborne and Mendel and McCollum and Davis, were also studying the effect of food on the health and growth of rats. Like Hopkins, they found that rats could not be kept alive on a diet of purified foods but that, with the addition of a small amount of milk, growth was normal. They suggested there were two factors in the milk; one in the fat of the milk which they called *Fat Soluble A* and one in the water of the milk which they called *Water Soluble B*.

Funk, a Polish chemist, thought the accessory food factors were protein in character and suggested the name *vitamines*. The first part of the name meant "vital" and the second part was derived from "amino-acids" of which proteins are formed. We know now that these accessory food factors are not protein in character at all. The name has, however, remained, but without the final "e" and we speak of *vitamin A, vitamin B, vitamin C,* and so on. The use of these letters is no longer really necessary since the chemical composition of all common vitamins has been determined. Each such vitamin has now been given its proper chemical name.

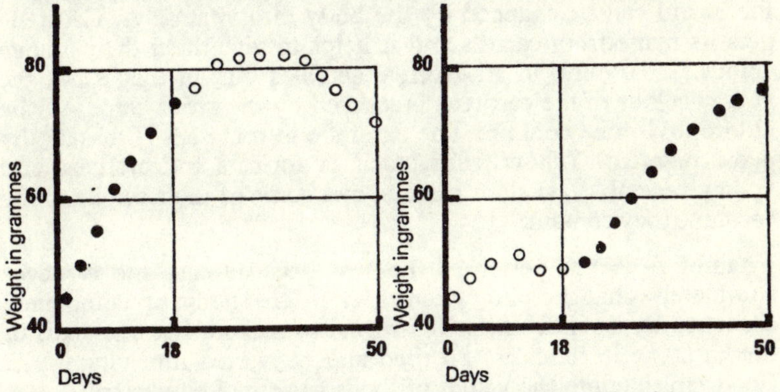

Graph of animal growth. Left-hand graph shows growth with vitamins (solid dots) to 18th day and decrease afterwards in absence of vitamins. Right-hand shows failure of growth in absence of vitamins and restoration of growth after the addition of vitamins to the diet.

The various vitamins are all distinct chemically. Each one plays a particular role in maintaining the processes of life and no one vitamin is able to do the work of another. It is, however, convenient to study them together for they are all organic (carbon-containing) substances which are required by the body, though in very small amounts, if it is to function properly.

Their function is the control of such bodily activities as growth, tissue repair and energy production. The body is unable to form vitamins for itself and must obtain them from food. They are present in foods in such small amounts that it is not surprising that their discovery has been so recent.

Lack of any one of the vitamins in the diet will lead to ill-health.

In serious cases, *deficiency diseases*, such as scurvy, beri-beri, pellagra and rickets are caused. Prolonged lack of vitamins may lead ultimately to death.

Vitamin A, Fat-Soluble A, Retinol, Axerophthol, Anti-infective Vitamin

Vitamin A is found in certain animal fats and in the fatty parts of some animal foods. Vegetable fats and oils contain little or no vitamin A.

A yellow substance, known as *carotene*, is found in certain vegetable foods and can be changed by the body into vitamin A. Carotene gets its name from carrots and it helps to give them their orange colour. It is found in all green vegetables but, in their case, the yellow colour of the carotene is masked by the green colour of the chlorophyll they contain. The carotene in tomatoes is masked by a red pigment. Yellow fruits, such as apricots and oranges, and yellow vegetables, such as carrots, owe some of their colour to the carotene they contain.

Vitamin A is the better of the two because carotene is never completely changed into vitamin A in the body or completely absorbed by the intestines. It is usual to reckon that one-sixth of the carotene in foods is absorbed and converted into vitamin A. Food tables quote the values of foods as retinol equivalents.

Vitamin A serves several purposes in the body:

(1) It is necessary for the growth of children.
(2) It helps the eye to perceive light.
(3) It protects the skin and ensures the activity of mucous membranes generally such as in the front of the eyes and the linings of the throat, bronchial tubes, stomach and intestines.

Lack of sufficient vitamin A checks the growth of children, particularly the correct growth of the bones and teeth. It also leads to inability to see well in a dim light and, in serious cases, to *night-blindness* as the vitamin is converted into the pigment visual purple which is present in the retina of the eye and is concerned with dim-light vision. Long continued deficiency of vitamin A leads to an eye disease known as *xerophthalmia* and ultimately to blindness.

The mucous membranes lining the throat and bronchial tubes and the outside (epithelial) linings of many glands and organs quickly become unhealthy and lose their power of secreting the lubricating mucus when vitamin A is lacking in the diet. In this unhealthy condition they offer lowered resistance to disease bacteria and the body is thus more easily infected with disease. This applies particularly to the organisms which cause the common cold and other diseases of the respiratory organs. Vitamin A is sometimes referred to as the *anti-infective vitamin*.

FOODS RICH IN VITAMIN A

Foods which contain vitamin A are fish liver oils, fat fish, liver and kidney, and dairy products—milk, cream, butter, cheese and egg yolk. Carotene is found in green vegetables, e.g., spinach, water-cress, cabbage and green peas; in yellow vegetables, e.g., carrots; and in apricots, tomatoes and yellow melons.

In the green vegetables the darker the green the more carotene will probably be present. The outer green leaves of cabbage, for example, are a good source of carotene while the inner white leaves of the heart contain none.

The vitamin A in milk, cream, butter and cheese has been formed by cows from the carotene in the green grass they have eaten. Summer milk and butter are thus better sources of vitamin A than winter milk and butter, and for the same reason New Zealand butter is particularly valuable in our winter.

Vitamin A finds its way into fat fish and fish liver from the minute green plants floating on the surface of the sea known as *plankton*. Small fish feed on this plankton and convert its carotene into vitamin A. Large fish eat the small fish and store up the vitamin A in their body oils and livers. This explains why halibut liver oil and cod liver oil are such excellent sources of vitamin A.

Vitamin A is soluble in fats, hence the old name, *fat-soluble vitamin A*. Both vitamin A and carotene are insoluble in water. Consequently, they are not leached out when foods containing them are soaked, boiled or steamed. Boiled carrots and cabbages contain just as much carotene as raw carrots and raw cabbages and are more easily digested.

The temperatures used for cooking are not likely to destroy the vitamin A and carotene in foods. Canned fruits and vegetables still contain their original carotene, and condensed and dried milk their original vitamin A.

We can store up vitamin A in the liver and so can utilise the excess supplies of one day to balance days when supplies are short. Plentiful summer supplies may carry us well into the winter when vitamin A is more difficult to obtain because greens and fruits are not so readily available. Deficiency of vitamin A takes several months to develop.

Since milk and butter contain less vitamin A in winter when dairy herds are largely fed on hay and mostly kept indoors and since green vegetables are scarce and expensive, foods such as liver, fat fish and carrots are particularly valuable during the period from September to April. Young children and nursing mothers who need additional amounts of vitamin A should supplement their supplies by taking halibut or cod liver oil.

Vegetable fats and oils are devoid of vitamin A. Margarines made from such fats and oils now have vitamin A added to them so as to make them equivalent in this respect to butter. The value is now 800–1000 μg per 100 g or 0·8–1·0 mg per 100 g.

The original way of measuring the effectiveness of vitamin A was by international units (i.u.). The new way is to use micrograms (μg) 2500 i.u. are equivalent to 750 μg.

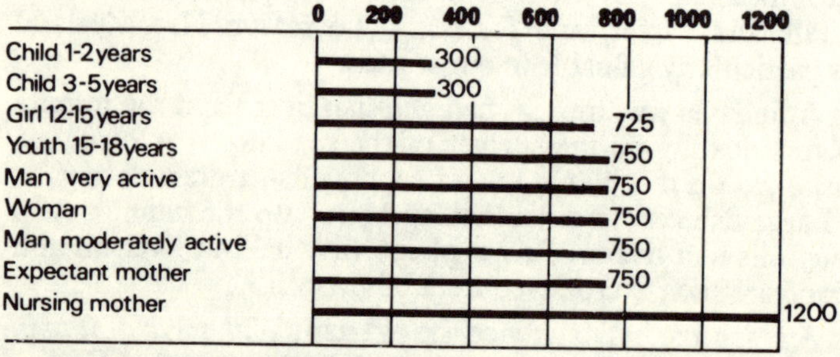

Vitamin A and carotene requirements as retinol equivalents in μg per day.

Vitamin B, Water-Soluble B, The Vitamin B Complex

The original water-soluble B factor has been found to be a mixture of several different vitamins which were numbered B_1, B_2 and so on, as they were discovered. Most of them now have their own chemical names and the whole collection of them (at least eleven) is known as the *vitamin B complex*. All are soluble in water and are usually, but not always, found together in the same foods. The body is unable to store these vitamins because of their solubility in water and, consequently, we need some every day.

It is only necessary for us to study three of the vitamins in the vitamin B complex. They are *thiamine*, *riboflavin* and *nicotinic acid*.

Vitamin B_1, Thiamine, Anti Beri-Beri or Anti-neuritic Vitamin

This vitamin is a white crystalline substance. It used to be known as *aneurine* (anti-neuritic vitamin) and its original name was *vitamin* B_1.

The function of thiamine in the body is to control the liberation of energy from carbohydrate foods by way of complete oxidation of glucose in the system. If thiamine is absent the glucose is incompletely oxidised and pyruvic acid is formed which damages the nerves.

Lack of thiamine in the diet leads to:

(1) A check in the growth of children.
(2) Loss of appetite, depression, fatigue, indigestion and constipation.
(3) Nervous irritability and a special type of neuritis (inflammation of the nerves).
(4) Prolonged deficiency leads to the disease beri-beri.

Beri-beri is a disease of the nervous system which causes a special type of paralysis. It is found chiefly in the Far East in such countries as Japan, the Malay Peninsula and the Dutch East Indies where most of the poor people live very largely on a diet of polished white rice. Natural unpolished rice contains thiamine in the outer "silver skin," or bran layer, which is removed during the preparation of polished rice.

The same loss of thiamine takes place when the bran layers and germ of wheat are removed in the milling of white flour. As with rice, the thiamine of wheat is found in the outside bran layers and the germ. True wholemeal flour, 100% extraction rate, contains all the thiamine of the original wheat. By Government Regulations all other types of flour must have thiamine added to them to compensate for that lost during milling. (See page 72.)

FOODS CONTAINING THIAMINE

Thiamine is widely distributed among foods but nearly always in small amounts. Important sources are whole grains; wholemeal and white flour and bread; oatmeal; dried brewers' yeast and yeast extracts; certain vegetables, especially legumes and potatoes; nuts; lean meat; pork and bacon; liver; fish roes; eggs; fish and milk. Bemax and Marmite are proprietary articles rich in thiamine prepared from wheat germ and yeast respectively, and most modern meat extracts are reinforced with the B vitamins.

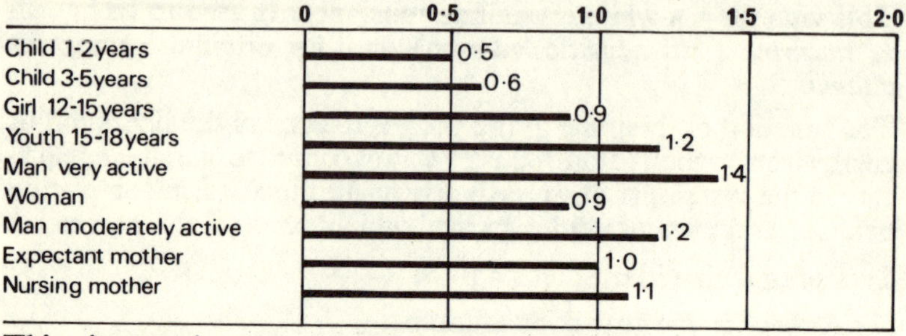

Thiamine requirements in milligrammes per day.

There are bacteria in the large intestine which can manufacture thiamine and some of this thiamine may pass into the blood stream and supplements that obtained from food.

Because thiamine is concerned with the metabolism of carbohydrate the amount of the vitamin needed bears a direct relationship to the amount of carbohydrate being used by the body. Therefore, for instance, people eating a large amount of carbohydrate food and engaged in heavy work will require more thiamine than people on a low carbohydrate diet engaged in light work.

By eating a good mixed diet containing plenty of natural foodstuffs, particularly wholegrain cereals, meats, milk and eggs, we should be able to meet our daily requirements easily. It is only when the diet is restricted too largely to highly refined carbohydrate foods such as polished rice and sugar that a deficiency of thiamine is likely to occur with consequent disorders of digestion and nervous tone. A deficiency of thiamine is very unlikely in this country.

Thiamine is very soluble in water and nearly half goes into the water in which fruits and vegetables are cooked. Between 20–40% of the vitamin is lost during the cooking.

Thiamine is destroyed by high temperatures. Meat loses 30–40% of the thiamine during roasting and stewing and there is a loss in the canning of meat and in the processing of foods where high temperatures are used. Temperatures reached in pressure cooking are likely to result in some loss of this vitamin.

Sodium bicarbonate destroys thiamine, and therefore the use of sodium bicarbonate to soften green vegetables and to give them a rich green colour will result in the destruction of the thiamine they contain; similarly the sodium bicarbonate used to make soda bread and scones will destroy much of the thiamine present.

The sulphites used as preservatives in sausages and in some canned meats have a similar effect upon the thiamine of the meat.

Vitamin B_2, Riboflavin

Riboflavin is the chemical name for the vitamin which was originally called B_2 in England. It is a greenish yellow substance which gives its characteristic colour to butter milk. It is concerned in the system with the production of energy by oxidation and also with the utilisation of food fats and amino-acids.

The symptoms of insufficient riboflavin in the diet are:

(1) A check in the growth of children.
(2) Inflammation of the mouth and tongue.
(3) The transparent front of the eye (the cornea) may become misted and vision be impaired.

FOODS CONTAINING RIBOFLAVIN

Riboflavin is not as widely distributed as thiamine but is found in much larger amounts in milk and milk products. Important sources are dried brewers' yeast, liver, meat and meat extracts,

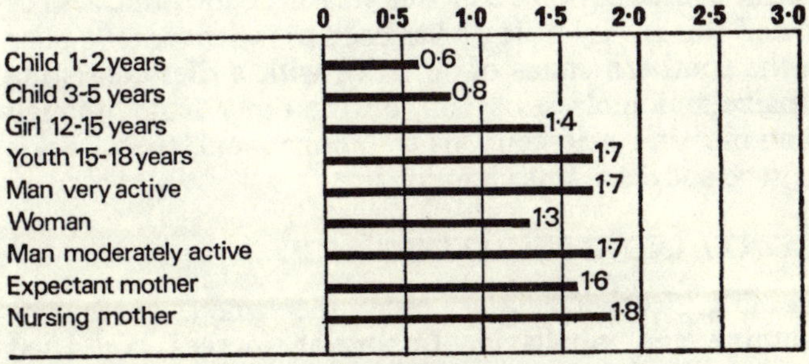

Riboflavin requirements in milligrammes per day.

cheese, eggs, pulses, nuts, milk and milk products, fish. Bemax and Marmite contain large amounts, beer contains useful amounts. There is little likelihood of a deficiency of riboflavin in a mixed diet in this country.

Because it is soluble, some of the riboflavin in foods is dissolved out when they are cooked in water. Very little is destroyed during ordinary boiling but losses do occur during frying, roasting and canning because of the high temperatures reached. There is a loss of riboflavin in milk left exposed to sunlight.

Nicotinic Acid, Niacin, Anti-pellagra Vitamin

Nicotinic acid is a white crystalline solid which is chemically allied to the nicotine of tobacco; hence the name. Nicotine is not a vitamin, but a dangerous poison and cannot be converted into nicotinic acid. The alternative name, *niacin*, is sometimes used to avoid confusion, especially in the U.S.A.

Its function in the body, like that of the other B-vitamins, is to help in the release of energy from carbohydrate foods.

Shortage of nicotinic acid causes:

(1) A check in the growth of children.
(2) Rough red skin and soreness of the tongue.
(3) Diarrhoea and other digestive troubles.
(4) In extreme cases, mental disorders and dementia.
(5) Finally, the disease pellagra and ultimately, death.

Nicotinic acid is converted in the body to an active form, known as nicotinamide, which is also formed from one of the amino-acids, tryptophan. Hence the body's needs may be obtained from either or both of these sources. Maize contains very little nicotinic acid or tryptophan and this is why pellagra has been prevalent among poor negroes in the southern states of America with a diet consisting largely of maize and molasses. Milk, on the other hand, though it contains no nicotinic acid contains tryptophan and, therefore, is indirectly a good source of this vitamin.

FOODS CONTAINING NICOTINIC ACID

Foods containing nicotinic acid are much the same as those containing thiamine and riboflavin. Important sources are dried brewers' yeast and yeast extracts; lean meat and meat extracts;

liver and kidney; white flour and bread; herrings and white fish; vegetables, particularly potatoes. Bemax and Marmite contain large amounts.

Sometimes nicotinic acid is present in a complex form, and it is then considered to be totally unavailable, as the complex molecule cannot be broken down to release the vitamin. Cereals, which used to be thought of as a good source of nicotinic acid, contain the vitamin in this complex form and so cannot be considered as a good source, though they do contribute towards the intake as they contain tryptophan.

Fortunately nicotinic acid is added to all white flour in Britain and this nicotinic acid, is, of course, available.

Nicotinic acid is very stable and there is no loss in cooking except that some is dissolved into the cooking water.

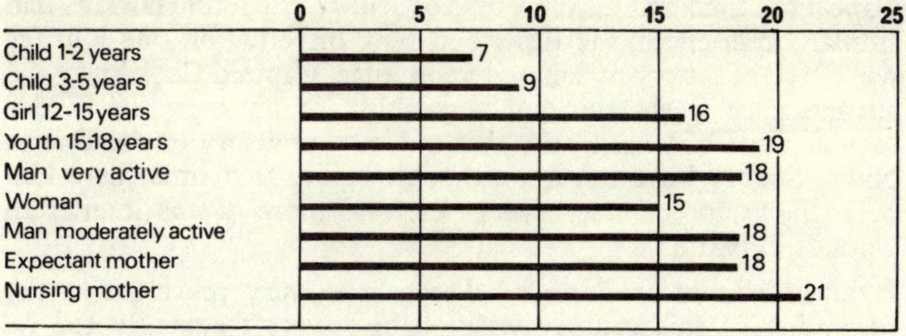

Nicotinic acid requirements in milligrammes per day.

Vitamin C, Ascorbic Acid, Anti-scorbutic Vitamin

Vitamin C is a white crystalline substance. Its chemical name, *ascorbic acid*, means the anti-scorbutic acid. Scorbutus is the medical name for the disease *scurvy*.

Ascorbic acid is needed for buoyant health, vitality and endurance. It ensures a clear skin, a fresh complexion and healthy gums and teeth.

Lack of ascorbic acid in the diet leads to:

(1) A check in the growth of children.
(2) Gums and teeth being easily infected.
(3) Slow healing of wounds and fractures.
(4) The disease, scurvy, in severe cases.

E

Scurvy is not simply a skin disease as most people imagine. It affects the whole system, particularly the blood vessels, gums, teeth and bones. The first symptoms of the disease are soreness of the gums and pains in the joints, e.g., the "growing pains" of quickly growing boys and girls. Later, the gums may become swollen and painful, the teeth become loose, the skin show bruise-like patches and the pains in the joints become unbearable. In extreme cases, the disease ends fatally unless stopped by an improvement in the diet.

Today the disease is rarely seen except in cases of unnaturally restricted diets such as may occur during explorations, sieges and famines. In the days of the old sailing ships scurvy was a veritable scourge among the sailors whose diet consisted mainly of salted meat and biscuits. Any kind of fresh fruit or vegetables was unheard of on board. During Vasco da Gama's voyage round the Cape more than half his crew died of scurvy. Sir John Hawkins had similar experiences. He described how his crew on one journey was cured of scurvy by taking lemon juice. Captain Cook knew the advantage of fresh fruit and vegetables for his crew. In 1795 a regular issue of lemon juice was made compulsory in the British Navy. Scurvy became rare, although before that time there had been thousands of cases every year and more deaths than from wounds in battle.

Infantile scurvy or Barlow's disease was very prevalent at the beginning of this century when babies were frequently fed on artificial baby foods without the addition of fruit juice. It is now common practice to give all babies orange juice daily.

Slight deficiencies are still found fairly frequently, for, as will be explained later, this vitamin is not present in many foods and is very easily destroyed during their preparation and cooking, so that people who live on a diet of sandwiches and snacks, or reheated meals, may well not have adequate supplies. For these people the only deficiency symptoms will be that their health will not be as good as it should be!

FOODS CONTAINING ASCORBIC ACID

We obtain our supplies of ascorbic acid from fruits and vegetables but not all fruits and vegetables are good sources. The best are soft summer fruits, e.g., blackcurrants, gooseberries, strawberries, raspberries and tomatoes; citrus fruits, e.g., oranges, lemons and grapefruits; green vegetables, e.g., cabbages, cauliflowers and sprouts; root vegetables, e.g., swedes and turnips; salad vegetables, e.g., watercress and mustard and cress. Although the potato does not contain a relatively large amount of ascorbic acid we eat so much of it and so regularly that it is one of our most valuable sources of supply. It is important to remember that cherries, plums, grapes, pears, apples (except Bramley's seedlings), carrots, lettuce and celery, contain very little ascorbic acid.

Seeds, including the cereals and dried peas and beans, contain no ascorbic acid (but it is formed in them if they are soaked in water and then sprouted for a few days). Among animal foods the only one to contain it is fresh liver, which contains a useful amount. Cow's milk contains small amounts only. Milk-fed babies need further supplies as from orange juice.

Blackcurrant syrup and purée, concentrated orange juice and rose hip syrup are useful supplements for infants, young children, expectant and nursing mothers, all of whom need extra amounts of ascorbic acid. Invalids, convalescents and persons who have had fractured limbs or operations are other examples of individuals needing additional supplies of this vitamin.

If we have good helpings of freshly cooked potatoes and of lightly cooked green vegetables, or swedes or a good helping of raw salad; or an orange or two tomatoes each day, we are not likely to suffer from lack of ascorbic acid. Contrary to general belief, "an apple a day" gives very little vitamin of any sort.

There are several difficulties that arise when one tries to ensure an adequate supply of vitamin C:

(1) The home-grown foods that supply the vitamin are mostly summer grown and so there is a seasonal glut followed by a shortage. This has been partly overcome by the importing of foods from abroad and by the much improved methods of preservation, in particular the development of deep-freezing.

(2) The vitamin is slowly destroyed by the normal activity of the plant cell enzymes, so that during storage particularly of vegetables there is a loss of the vitamin. (Destruction of the vitamin in acid fruits is prevented by the presence of the fruit acid.) Thus potatoes, which can be considered as a good source of vitamin C in the autumn, gradually lose the vitamin so that by, say, March there is very little of the vitamin left.

(3) Ascorbic acid is very readily destroyed by the oxygen of the air. Therefore if air can enter the cell it will destroy any Vitamin C present. Air may either get into the cell when water is lost on wilting, or when the cell wall is damaged. It is therefore important to use vegetables soon after they have been picked and before they have had time to wilt. One must also try to keep damage to a minimum and this includes damage done during the preparation of the food for the table.

(4) Vitamin C is destroyed by heat. The higher the temperature, and the longer it goes on the greater the destruction of the vitamin.

(5) Vitamin C is extremely soluble in water and can very easily be washed out of the food during cooking.

Fortunately there are various things which can help in the retention of the vitamin. Freezing will reduce the activity of the enzymes and the rate of oxidation and so help to reduce the rate of loss of the vitamin. Heat will destroy the enzymes and so prevent their activity (but see 4 above). Acids, including the acids of fruit, will help to preserve Vitamin C against destruction by both air and enzymes. And lastly although the vitamin is extremely soluble in water, if one uses the water that the food has been cooked in then one is retaining the dissolved vitamin.

Thus when fruit and vegetables are cooked, ascorbic acid is lost by way of heat, and of enzymes, and of its solution in the water in which they are soaked or cooked. These losses can be reduced to a minimum by:

(1) Using fruit and vegetables as fresh as possible.
(2) Storing in a cool damp place.
(3) Avoiding crushing or bruising.
(4) Avoiding soaking whenever possible and never soaking for long.
(5) Coarsely shredding vegetables and immediately placing them in the smallest possible quantity of boiling water.
(6) Boiling with the lid on the pan so as to reduce the rate of oxidation.
(7) Dishing up and serving immediately after cooking.
(8) Using the cooking water for soups, stews and gravies.

However, it is unfortunately impossible to avoid some loss and this is likely to be about 50% of the content of the green leafy vegetables and about 30% of potatoes.

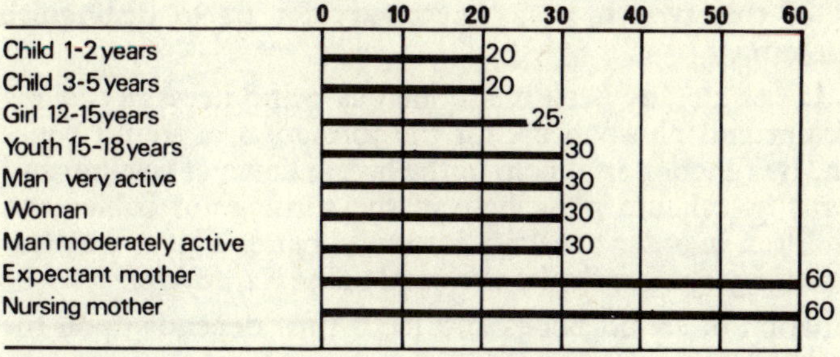

Ascorbic acid requirements in milligrammes per day.

The addition of soda to green vegetables to soften them and preserve their colour destroys vitamin B_1, and vitamin C. Keeping potatoes and greens hot for a long time after cooking, or reheating after standing, as often happens in canteens and restaurants, is very definitely destructive of any ascorbic acid they may still contain and should be avoided whenever possible.

Commercially canned fruits and vegetables, when modern methods are used, will have a higher ascorbic acid content than the correspondingly incorrectly home-cooked foods. The bottling of vegetables is less likely to successfully preserve the vitamin but much of the vitamin of bottled fruit is preserved. Recent improved methods of dehydrating vegetables have resulted in much smaller losses of ascorbic acid than was the case with older methods and as much vitamin is present in a serving of cooked dehydrated cabbage as in a similar portion of freshly cooked cabbage. Deep-frozen foods retain much of their ascorbic acid and if correctly stored and prepared will supply as much of the vitamin as the fresh food would have done.

Jams and marmalades still retain some of the ascorbic acid of the original fruits; how much depends upon the circumstances of picking, storage and preparation.

All these points about ascorbic acid have been emphasised because, of all the vitamins we require, it is the one most likely to be deficient in the average diet in this country.

Vitamin D, Calciferol, Calcifying Vitamin, Sunshine Vitamin, Anti-rachitic Vitamin

Strictly speaking there is more than one vitamin D but in a

textbook of this type it is not necessary for us to distinguish between them.

Vitamin D has already been mentioned as being necessary, along with calcium and phosphorus, for the formation of sound bones and teeth. Its function is to help in the laying down of calcium and phosphorus as calcium phosphate in the cartilage of babies and young children in order to calcify it to solid bone. This is why it is called the *calcifying vitamin*. Its chemical name is *calciferol*.

The formation of sound bones and teeth thus depends upon the body receiving:

(1) Sufficient calcium in the diet.
(2) Sufficient phosphorus in the diet.
(3) Calcium and phosphorus in the right proportion to each other.
(4) Sufficient vitamin D in the diet.

If one or other of calcium, phosphorus or vitamin D is insufficient, or if the calcium and phosphorus are in the wrong proportions, then the disease *rickets*, in some greater or less degree, occurs. In extreme cases, the bones remain soft and bend easily thus leading to bow legs and knock-knees and swollen wrists and ankles. Until quite recently, rickets was very common in this country, particularly among the poorer people in thickly populated industrial areas. In fact, it is still known on the Continent as the "English disease". Fortunately, it is much less common at the present time and now that the cause is known it should never occur again. Because of its role in the prevention of rickets, vitamin D is sometimes referred to as the *anti-rachitic* (*anti-rickets*) *vitamin*.

Infants and young children, expectant and nursing mothers have the greatest need of vitamin D but adults require a small amount.

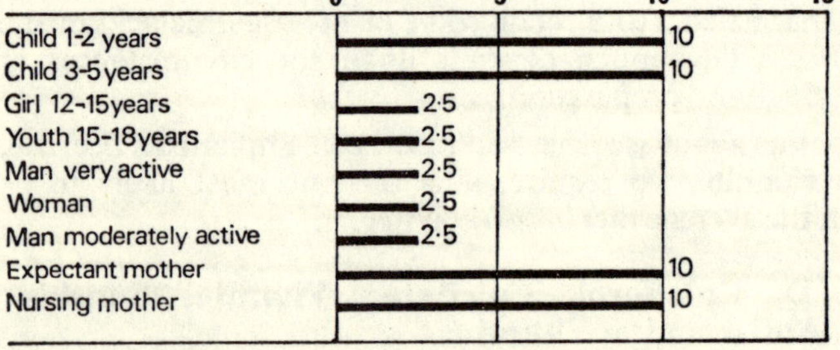

Vitamin D requirements in microgrammes per day.

The exact amount of vitamin needed is difficult to determine because sunlight can convert ergosterol in the skin to Vitamin D (see below). However the amounts given here appear adequate to ensure enough of the vitamin even for those who spend most of their time indoors. The older unit for measuring Vitamin D has now been replaced by the microgram. 1 $\mu g = 40$ international units (i.u.). When the diet of an adult is deficient in calcium, phosphorus or vitamin D, a disease of the bones similar to rickets may occur. It is known as *osteomalacia*.

FOODS CONTAINING VITAMIN D

Very few foods contain vitamin D and, with very few exceptions, they are animal foods. Those which contain most are halibut liver oil, cod liver oil; herrings, mackerel, sardines and salmon; eggs, butter, cheese, vitaminised margarine and milk. In other words, they are fish liver oils, fat fish and dairy foods.

The fat fish are much richer sources of vitamin D than the dairy foods; halibut liver oil and cod liver oil contain very much larger quantities still. Unfortunately the taste of these fish liver oils is obnoxious to most people. Young children, however, if started early enough, can be trained not only to take them but actually to relish them. Failing this they can be given in the form of capsules or their taste masked in fish sauces, soups, mayonnaise, savouries, and so on.

The supply of vitamin D from foods can be supplemented by the body itself in a most interesting way. Underneath the skin is a layer of fat which contains a fat-like substance called *ergosterol*. When the body is exposed to bright summer or mountain sunshine this substance is converted into vitamin D which the body is able to store and to utilise. It is the powerful ultra-violet rays of the sun which bring about this change. The rays given out by special mercury vapour lamps ("sun ray" lamps) similarly produce vitamin D under the skin. Clinics and hospitals use them to assist in the cure of rickets. These ultra-violet lamps can also be used to convert the ergosterol of food into vitamin D. The food is then described as "irradiated".

The formation of vitamin D from ergosterol by sunlight explains why rickets is seldom seen in hot tropical countries except where the purdah system is in operation and women and children are confined indoors. It explains why in our climate rickets was more common among the poorer children living in overcrowded conditions in smoky industrial towns, and why it is sometimes seen today in immigrant Asian children and in the housebound elderly. All such groups may receive little vitamin D from their diet and have little exposure to sunshine. It is an interesting fact that rickets is rare among Eskimos. They get very little sunshine but they live largely on fish.

Infants and expectant and nursing mothers need more vitamin D than others and should have halibut liver oil or cod liver oil daily. The rest of us should eat fat fish regularly, get out into the midday sunshine whenever possible, and have our summer holidays at the seaside.

Like vitamin A, vitamin D is not soluble in water but is soluble in fats and consequently can be stored in the fats of the body. The two vitamins usually occur together in the same foods. Vitamin D is not lost in cooking water or destroyed by the heat of cooking. Modern margarines have vitamin D as well as vitamin A added to them.

Other vitamins, not mentioned here, are just as important as these ones. But, generally, if the diet is satisfactory in the nutrients so far detailed, then there will be satisfactory supplies of all nutrients.

PART TWO

7 The Cereals

The term "cereals" includes wheat, oats, barley, rye, rice and maize. Sometimes the term is widened to include sago, tapioca and arrowroot which are not cereals at all, and sometimes narrowed to mean the specially prepared foods frequently eaten at breakfast. Strictly speaking, cereals are cultivated grasses. It is the seeds of these cultivated grasses with their rich storehouses of food for the young plants which we eat.

They are the most important of all plant foods. We eat more cereal food than any other. It is no exaggeration to say that without cereals modern civilisation would be impossible. Cereals are easily cultivated, can be conveniently transported and stored in bulk for long periods. They are palatable, cheap and readily prepared for the table. There are few parts of the world where a cereal of some type cannot be grown. For these reasons, man has been able to adopt a settled communal life, first in crude homesteads and settlements and finally in cities, instead of the nomadic life he would have had to follow had he remained dependent upon flocks and herds for his food. In the Lord's Prayer bread is taken as symbolical of food and we often refer to bread as "the staff of life." Cereals are the principal food of mankind and bread—usually made from wheat—is the staple article of diet for millions of human beings.

By centuries of cultivation and selection the original wild grass seeds have become modified and developed until their food value has been greatly increased and their yield multiplied. They are still, however, far from perfect foods. Though they contain a fair amount of protein (7·2% rice to 13% oats) yet its biological value is inferior to that of most animal proteins.

However, because cereals make up such a large proportion of our diet, they supply us with quite a large part of our total protein. They contain only small quantities of fat (1·7% wheat to 8·1% oats) and are deficient in vitamins A, C and D. Their content of the B group of vitamins depends upon the degree and type of milling to which they have been subjected. Certain minerals, notably calcium, phosphorus and iron, are also deficient and their availability is affected by the presence of phytic acid which makes them insoluble. The amount of carbohydrate in the whole grain varies from 59% in oats to 79% in rice, mainly in the form of starch.

Cereals are thus principally sources of carbohydrate and are therefore mainly energy foods. They provide the largest proportion of the energy value of the diet for most of mankind. The great preponderance of starch in cereals makes it necessary to eat them along with foods rich in protein and fat, and this we do when we make puddings with eggs and milk and eat bread with butter or cheese.

Compared with other plant foods, the amounts of moisture in cereal grains are small, varying from 7% in oats to 12% in wheat. This makes them very compact foods and accounts for their keeping qualities. The indigestible part of cereal grains is almost entirely confined to the outside skin layers. When this is removed during milling the starch which is left is easily digested.

WHEAT

So far as we are concerned in this country, wheat is the most important of the cereals just as, for climatic reasons, rice is the main food cereal of the Chinese and Japanese. This is fortunate for us because wheat is undoubtedly the king of the cereals. Compared with other cereals, its protein content is high and, when mixed with water, wheat flour forms an elastic, tenacious dough which can be aerated and made into a light, porous, palatable bread. It is impossible to make bread of the same character from rice, oats, barley, rye or maize. Unlike wheat, none contains sufficient of the protein, gluten, which combines with water to form a dough.

Wheat was probably first grown in Mesopotamia and Egypt and was originally a sub-tropical plant. Varieties of wheat have now been produced which can be cultivated from the tropics to the very edge of the Arctic Circle. Some varieties can resist drought, others can withstand cold. The regions where wheat cultivation is most extensively practised are shown on the map of the world.

The many varieties of wheat can be divided into two main classes, winter wheat and spring wheat. Different areas of the world, according to their climates, grow either one type or the other. Winter wheat is sown in the autumn and, after germination and some growth, the young plant stays almost dormant until early spring. It is harvested in the following autumn. In regions where the soil is frozen for long periods in the winter, spring wheat must be grown. This is sown and harvested in the same year and a hot dry summer is necessary for it to ripen. In this country we grow chiefly winter wheat: Argentina, Canada, U.S.A., the Soviet Union and the Danubian countries grow spring wheat.

Winter wheat, with its long growing period in temperate climates, produces a "soft" flour with a good flavour but with only low gluten content. This flour forms a weak dough and bakes into

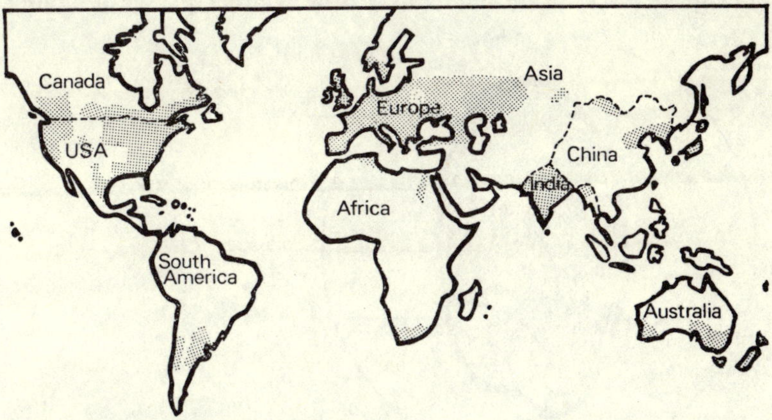

Wheat-producing areas of the world.

small loaves of close texture. Spring wheat, ripened in hot dry summers, produces a "strong" flour with a harsh flavour but rich in gluten so that it forms a strong dough and bakes into well-risen and shapely loaves. Strong flour is also used for the manufacture of "pasta", the "macaroni-type" products so extensively used in Italy where the wheat has a high gluten content. Because of the differences in gluten content, flours of the different types are usually blended by the miller to make them suitable for particular purposes. The doughs of strong flours are difficult to work by hand but are very suitable for large-scale machine breadmaking. Soft flours are more suitable for household cooking, cakes and biscuits.

THE STRUCTURE OF THE WHEAT GRAIN

A spike of ripe wheat consists of a stalk to which the wheat grains or "berries" are attached and each grain is covered by a protective yellow leaf or glume. When the wheat is threshed the grain is separated from the stalk and glumes that form straw and chaff respectively. The berries themselves are roughly barrel-shaped and more pointed at one end than the other. At the pointed end is a small tuft of hairs, known as the "beard," and at the blunt end, which was originally attached to the stalk, is a small rough protuberance. This is the wheat embryo—the living part of the grain from which, on germination, the seedling develops. On one side a deep crease or furrow passes along the whole length of the grain. The grain is split open along this furrow in an early stage of milling.

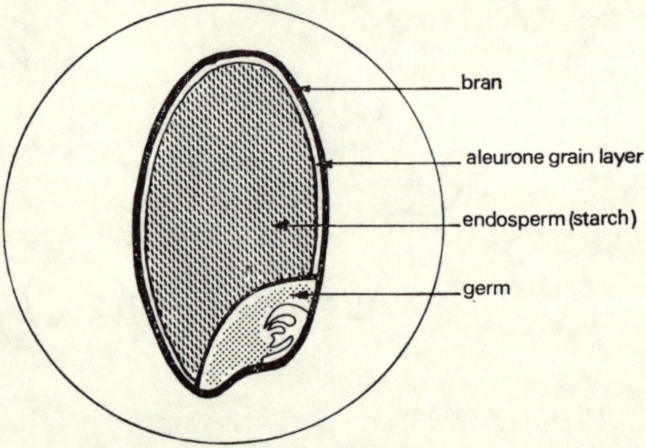

Longitudinal section of a wheat grain.

The wheat grain is the fruit of the plant. Fruits in general contain a seed or seeds surrounded by a protective covering known as the seed coat or testa and the whole is enclosed in an outer fruit wall or pericarp. In the case of the wheat plant, the fruit consists of a single seed with both testa and pericarp closely attached to one another. In the milling of wheat these outside skins, which consist of cellulose impregnated with mineral matter, constitute the bran or "offal." They form about 13% by weight of the whole grain.

Underneath the pericarp comes the layer of roughly cubical cells known as the aleurone layer. The aleurone cells are packed with protein granules and contain also nicotinic acid, iron and enzymes. In spite of its food value the miller excludes this layer from white flour along with the outside bran layers since it is apt to spoil its keeping and baking qualities.

The rest of the berry consists of the endosperm and the germ or embryo. The endosperm is packed with starch grains with the spaces between them filled with the protein, gluten. The endosperm is much the largest part of the wheat grain and makes up about 85% of its weight. It is the embryo's storehouse of food and is the part of the wheat berry which the miller makes into white flour.

The embryo or germ lies to the base of the endosperm and is the living part of the berry. It consists of three parts—plumule, radicle and scutellum. Its weight is less than 2% of the whole grain. The plumule is the undeveloped shoot and the radicle the undeveloped root. The scutellum (or little shield) lies between the endosperm and the embryo proper, and contains the enzymes that can change the starch and gluten of the endosperm into soluble forms suitable as food for the embryo when it germinates. The embryo and scutellum contains most of the fat of the grain as well as some protein, calcium, iron and the vitamins thiamine, riboflavin and nicotinic acid. The fat and enzymes of the embryo affect the keeping quality of flour, for the fat is liable to turn rancid and the enzymes to attack the starch and gluten of the flour. For this reason it is excluded by the miller along with the bran or offal in the making of white flour, to be used for the feeding of cattle and poultry.

THE MILLING OF WHEAT

The outside skins of the wheat grain are so firmly attached to the endosperm that without some sort of preparation it is practically impossible to digest the whole grain. One old-fashioned method of using whole grains as food was to soak them in water until they burst and then gently to boil them in milk with the addition of sugar and sometimes dried fruit and spices as flavouring. This very nourishing dish was known as "frumenty." More modern and convenient methods are those of "shredding" or "puffing" such as are used in making some breakfast foods.

Usually, however, wheat before eating is reduced to a fine powdery flour by the process of grinding or milling. The old method was that of grinding the grains between flat grooved mill stones. All the parts of the grain were incorporated in a wholemeal flour. Sometimes the wholemeal was sifted through muslin to remove the coarser bran layers. This type of stone-ground flour retained the greater part of the nutritive value of the whole grain but it was dark in colour because of fine bran particles and did not keep well because it contained the fat and enzymes of the germ. It produced a dark, coarse and rather indigestible loaf which went stale quickly.

Modern roller milling involves a large number of complex processes which we can only describe very briefly. First the wheat is thoroughly cleaned by passing through a series of complicated machines which remove dust, soil, stones, weed seeds, chaff and so on. Next comes washing in cold water followed by drying, cooling and storing. The wheat grains are now perfectly clean with the outside bran layers toughened and the inside endosperm dry and brittle. Blending of different varieties of wheat now follows to give the type of flour required.

The next stage of the milling process is the passing of the grains through fluted rollers, one of which revolves more quickly than the other. The grains are split open at the crease and most of the endosperm is released. The outside skin layers are broken up into flakes. The mixture is sifted and the skin and coarser particles passed through further pairs of rollers until the remains of the endosperm are scraped off the skin. Finally the brittle particles of endosperm are passed through a series of smooth rollers which crush them to a fine powder. The tougher, oilier particles of germ are flattened out but not powdered so that in the final sieving through silk sieves they will not pass through while the flour will.

The flour is now stored for a period of several weeks and a process known as "aging" takes place, during which the oxygen of the air improves the elastic qualities of the gluten. Chemicals called "improvers" are usually added to hasten this process.

By this modern process of milling it is possible to produce a white flour consisting of practically nothing but the endosperm. Such a flour keeps well, bakes well and gives an attractive and easily digested white bread which does not go stale quickly. Its nutritive value, however, is less than that of stone-ground flour because of the removal of the aleurone layer, germ and scutellum, with their valuable B vitamins, protein and iron.

For a long time there has been controversy between millers and dietitians as to which is the best type of flour. The millers, on the one hand, prefer to produce a white flour containing only about 70% of the original grain (70% extraction), for such a flour keeps well and pleases the baker and the general public because of its baking qualities and the good appearance and digestibility of the loaf it produces. The bran or offal is used for feeding poultry, pigs and cattle. Unlike human beings, they can digest it and convert it into meat, eggs and milk. The germ is used in making special "germ" flours such as Hovis and proprietary foodstuffs such as Bemax.

On the other hand some dietitians argue that we ought to obtain the maximum food value from wheat by using a flour from which only the coarser particles of bran have been removed (95% extraction). In this way we obtain not only the ingredients of the endosperm but also the protein, fat, B vitamins, calcium and iron of the germ and aleurone layer. The particles of bran act as roughage, assist the peristaltic action of the intestines, and so help to prevent constipation.

In order to economise in valuable shipping space during World War II, the extraction rate was gradually increased from the 70% pre-war rate to 85% as the shipping shortage became more and more acute. By so doing a larger and larger proportion of the protein, fat, B vitamins, calcium and iron was included in the so-called "National" flour. Unfortunately, the inclusion of increased amounts of bran and germ meant that phytic acid, which is found mainly in the bran and germ, might make much of the calcium and iron of flour and other foods unavailable and thus antagonise the calcification of bones and teeth. The Ministry of Food took a serious view of this possibility since it was known that the pre-war British diet was short of calcium and in 1943 the addition of calcium to flour was made compulsory. This "fortification" (now 1 part chalk to 320 parts of flour) is still in operation although it is now known that much of the phytic acid in bread is broken down by yeast during baking.

In 1944 improved milling techniques made it possible to separate out the most nutritious parts of the germ and scutellum of the wheat and obtain a flour of 80% extraction which gave a loaf of highly satisfactory food value and, at the same time, a quite acceptable off-white colour, good flavour and good keeping

F

qualities. It represented a reasonable compromise between the competing claims of millers, farmers, bakers, housewives and dietitians.

In 1953 an extraction rate of under 80% became permissible and from that time onward the rate gradually fell until in 1956 it was reduced to the pre-war 70% with a consequent decrease in the amounts of thiamine, nicotinic acid and iron. In accordance with the Report of a Government Panel set up in 1956 to study the problem, all flours, except 100% extraction wholemeal, must have thiamine, nicotinic acid and iron (in addition to calcium) added to them to make them equivalent to the 80% "National" flour. The latest order brought into force in 1964 gives the following as the minimum quantities of nutrients that must be present in every 100 grammes of flour:

Iron 1·65 mg; Thiamine 0·24 mg; Nicotinic acid 1·60 mg.

Much of the calcium in wholemeal flour is not available as it is present as calcium phytate, and similarly the nicotinic acid of the cereal is not available, and so it is arguable that the modern white flour is nutritionally better in all respects except its protein content. The nutritive value of flour is a matter of great importance since bread and flour contribute about 26% thiamine, 22% iron, 13% nicotinic acid, 16% calcium and 19% protein in the average household diet.

SPECIAL FLOURS

Germ Meals

Quite a number of these are sold as proprietary articles. One of the best known, Hovis, is prepared by mixing 75% white flour with 25% cooked germ. Before adding to the white flour, the germ is mixed with the necessary amount of salt for breadmaking and then partly cooked by superheated steam. This pre-cooking produces a characteristic flavour and destroys the enzymes of the germ as well as preventing the oil of the germ from going rancid.

Self-raising Flours

These are simply ordinary flours with the necessary aerators added to them for confectionery purposes. The necessary proportions of, for example, cream of tartar and bicarbonate of soda are carefully sieved and dried and then thoroughly mixed with dry flour. Convenience is their only advantage.

Starch-reduced Flours

"Energen" rolls, made from flour which has had much of its starch washed out, and "Procea" bread, made from flour to which extra gluten has been added, can be purchased. Both products are much lighter and have a lower kilocalorie value than the same volume of ordinary bread. Since the amount of bread and rolls we eat is determined by volume rather than by weight, Energen rolls and Procea bread are often recommended in slimming diets. Eating less of ordinary bread would be equally effective.

WHEAT PRODUCTS

Semolina

Semolina is made from the central part of the endosperms of hard wheats rich in gluten. Some wheats of hot dry countries, such as France and Italy, are particularly suitable for its preparation. The grains are granulated into coarse particles by not crushing them sufficiently to reduce them completely to flour. Semolina is useful for making puddings and for thickening soups.

Macaroni, Vermicelli, Spaghetti and Italian Paste

These also are made from hard wheats grown in Italy, Southern Russia, and, more recently, Canada and U.S.A. The flour is made into a paste with water which, because of the large amount of gluten present, can be drawn into tubes or moulded into various shapes. The paste is afterwards dried and partly baked. They are mainly energy foods but they do contain more protein than normal flour and their nutritive value is greatly increased by the milk and flour eaten with them. Some pastas also have egg added during their manufacture. However, the flour used in the manufacture of pasta will not have had the extra calcium, iron, thiamine and nicotinic acid added that is added to British flour.

Shredded Wheat

Shredded wheat is made from the whole wheat grains in the form of shreds which have been cooked.

Force and Grape Nuts

These are malted whole wheat which has been cooked.

Puffed Wheat

Puffed wheat is made by cooking whole wheat grains in sealed ovens at a high temperature. When the pressure is released the grains swell up to many times their original size.

These breakfast foods are quickly prepared and easily digested but are a more expensive source of energy than either porridge or bread.

OATS

Oats have the highest food value of any of the cereals. Compared with the other cereals, they contain considerably more fat and have energy value. Their proteins are of higher biological value but do not include gluten so they do not form a dough with water and cannot be made into bread. A drawback is the presence of much phytic acid.

Oats are one of the hardiest cereals and can be grown in northerly latitudes unfavourable to wheat. It is for this reason that Scotland and the north of England grow large quantities of oats. Oats have for centuries been a staple article of diet in Scotland and until modern times were the main food of the workers of the north as in havercakes and porridge.

When milled for human consumption, oats are first cleaned from weed seeds, small stones, etc., and then kiln dried and stored for twenty-four hours before the closely adherent outside husk can be removed. In this form they are known as groats, which are ground to produce oatmeal. Rolled oats are made by partially cooking groats by steam before rolling them into flakes and drying them.

Oatmeal is usually eaten in the form of porridge or oatcakes. Rolled oats are more easily made into porridge than oatmeal because of their crushing and preliminary cooking. On account of the large amount of cellulose, oatmeal should always be thoroughly softened and well cooked, otherwise it will be indigestible. When combined with milk and sugar or syrup, porridge is an excellent food. The milk is particularly valuable in that its high proportion of calcium largely counterbalances the phytic acid of the oats which tends to make their calcium and iron unavailable. Cheese with oatcakes serves the same purpose.

Oatmeal is added to many meat and vegetable dishes and used to thicken soups and stews. If first toasted in the oven it may be used for coating fish cakes and rissoles. It may be added in small proportions to wheat flour in making pastry, scones, puddings, cakes and biscuits. It is a pity that so nutritious a cereal should be eaten less by human beings than by horses.

Because of its fat, oatmeal will not keep as well as wheat flour. It should be stored in a container with a tightly fitting lid and kept in a cool place.

BARLEY

Barley is the hardiest of all cereals and can thrive under climatic conditions that would not permit the survival of wheat. In spite of this, its use as a human food has steadily declined throughout the centuries and barley has now been superseded by wheat. It is probable that the "daily bread" of the Lord's Prayer was made from barley as well as the five loaves that fed the five thousand. Barley is now used mainly for the manufacture of malt for making beer and whisky and for stock feeding. Its only uses as human food are as barley water and for thickening soups. It cannot be made into a light spongy bread because of its lack of gluten.

"Pearl Barley" is made by polishing the kernel after the husk has been removed. "Scotch Barley" retains some of the husk layers. "Patent Barley" is pearl barley ground into flour.

Barley water, when flavoured with orange or lemon juice, makes a pleasant drink which has valuable demulcent properties.

RYE

Rye, like barley and oats, can grow under conditions unfavourable to wheat. It resembles wheat in its composition and contains a small amount of gluten which is sufficient to give an elastic dough with water capable of aeration by yeast, leaven or baking powder. Rye flour makes a dark, close, heavy bread with a sour flavour since it is usually aerated with sour dough (leaven). It is improved by mixing with a considerable proportion of wheat flour. Rye has been superseded in most parts of the world by wheat but is still a staple article of diet among the poorer people of Europe.

Ryvita is prepared from crushed whole rye.

RICE

Rice, the main cereal of the Orient, forms the staple article of food for nearly half the world's population. It requires a hot humid atmosphere, caused by heavy rains and hot sunshine, and needs irrigation in its early stages of growth. It is the only cereal that can be grown in many parts of the tropics.

Rice contains more starch than any of the other cereals but is the poorest in protein, fat and mineral matter. Since it is eaten in this country mainly in the form of rice puddings in which milk, fat and sugar are used this is of little consequence to us. Eggs and cheese are also valuable supplements to rice.

In the milling of rice, the bran and germ arc first removed and afterwards the silver skin underneath the bran is removed by polishing. As previously mentioned (page 51) the removal of the silver skin takes away the vitamin B_1 it contains and, where the diet consists largely of polished rice, beri-beri frequently occurs. We eat so little rice that it does not matter whether we eat it polished or unpolished, but it matters a great deal in predominantly rice-eating countries like India, Burma, Malaya, China and Japan. Attempts are being made to encourage the use of unpolished brown rice or polished rice which has been parboiled and dried before removing the bran, germ and silver skin. During the parboiling, sufficient of the soluble vitamin B_1 is absorbed by the endosperm to prevent beri-beri.

Besides being used whole, rice is used in this country as ground rice or rice flour in cakes, for the manufacture of puffed rice, and so on.

MAIZE

Maize originated in America where it is termed corn or Indian corn. It will flourish in any warm climate where there is summer rainfall. It does not require the swampy conditions necessary for rice. The wet summer suitable for maize is unsuitable for wheat.

The cultivation of maize has now spread to Mediterranean countries and Africa. In Italy a porridge, known as "polenta," is made from corn meal with the addition of cheese. In Africa, maize is called "mealies." Mealie pap, consisting mainly of maize with a little meat, forms the staple native diet.

Maize meal, or corn meal, is prepared by grinding after first removing the germ and husk. Hominy is less finely ground than corn meal and is in the form of hard gritty particles. Cornflour is essentially the crushed endosperm of the maize grain. The protein and fat are washed away so that cornflour consists almost entirely of starch. Cornflakes consist of cooked maize that has been dried, rolled and toasted.

The proteins of maize do not form a glutinous substance with water as do those of wheat, so that maize meal cannot be made into a spongy bread. Cornbreads are unleavened and flat. The fats of maize are next in amount to those of oats but are liable to go rancid and have a peculiar flavour. The small amount of nicotinic acid in maize renders persons eating a diet containing large amounts of maize liable to the disease pellagra. (See page 54.) Much of the nicotinic acid in maize is in the bound form, and maize only contains small amounts of the amino-acid, tryptophan, which acts as a precursor of nicotinic acid. However, where there is a good mixed diet the lack of nicotinic acid in maize is no great detriment.

We use it here as cornflour, in custard powders, blancmanges and sauces and as the breakfast food "Cornflakes." Occasionally, it is used as a vegetable. "Corn on the cob" is the green unripe head of the corn stalk and contains sugar rather than starch. Maize is highly esteemed in this form in America.

The starch of cornflour is particularly suitable for custard powders and blancmanges because it forms a paste that sets with a "short" texture and leaves the mould more cleanly than the pastes formed by the starches of wheat, potatoes, tapioca or arrowroot. Cornflour is a concentrated energy food and forms a vehicle for milk in blancmanges and custards.

SAGO, TAPIOCA AND ARROWROOT

These are not cereals, since they are not products of cultivated grasses, but it is convenient to consider them here. They contain practically no protein and are little more than refined preparations of starch.

Sago is produced from the pith of the sago palm.

Tapioca is derived from the roots of the tropical cassava plant after the removal of a bitter poisonous juice.

Arrowroot is obtained from the underground stem (rhizome) of the West Indian plant, maranta. It has the most delicate flavour of the three.

Since these preparations consist almost entirely of carbohydrate, they should not be eaten alone but with substances rich in protein, fat, minerals and vitamins. This is usually done by making them into puddings with milk and eggs. During the preparation of sago, tapioca and arrowroot many of the starch cells are burst and this makes them easily cooked and digestible.

8 Fats and Sugars

FATS

The chemical nature of fats and their purpose in the diet has already been fully discussed in Chapter 3. Cream, butter and margarine are described in the chapter on milk. It only remains here to give a few details about lard, suet, dripping and cooking fats.

Lard

Lard is the rendered fat from the fat deposits of pigs. It is practically 100% fat and consequently has a high energy value. Lard has a low melting point, a soft consistency and a pleasant, mild flavour. It is more easily digested than harder fats with higher melting points such as beef and mutton fats. Unlike the majority of animal fats it contains no vitamin A or D. Lard is used chiefly for pastry making and for shallow fat frying.

Suet

Suet is the fat round the internal organs of animals. It is a hard solid fat enclosed in connective tissue. Suet can be used finely chopped or, more usually, it is rendered, flaked and mixed with flour to prevent the flakes from sticking together. It can be used in a variety of ways and is a means of providing fat in the diet in a form acceptable to children and to those with an aversion to other forms of fat. Suet should be thoroughly cooked by boiling or steaming: otherwise it is indigestible.

Dripping

Dripping is the fat collected during the cooking of beef or mutton. It is usually brown in colour and is flavoured by the meat. Owing to the water and meat extracts it contains it is liable to go rancid if kept for too long. If used for frying or pastry making it may give a noticeable flavour unless purified by clarifying. This is done by putting the fat in a saucepan without lid, covering with water, bringing to the boil and pouring into a clean basin. When cold, the fat will form a hard cake on top of the water and any impurities will be either in the water or on the bottom of the fat. The cake of fat is lifted out, turned upside down and the bottom scraped clean. The fat is then suitable for pastry or puddings. For frying or keeping, the water it contains should be removed by melting it in a saucepan and heating it gently until it stops bubbling, i.e., until all the water has been driven out as steam.

Frying fats

These are made from whale oil and vegetable oils such as groundnut oil, cotton seed oil, coconut oil, palm kernel oil and palm oil.

In their natural forms these oils have a strong smell and taste, and do not keep well. They can be hardened by the process of hydrogenation into solid fats which keep well and are tasteless and odourless. In this process hot hydrogen gas is pumped into the oils in the presence of finely divided nickel which enables the oils to combine with the hydrogen gas.

To be suitable for making pastry, cakes and puddings, a fat should have a pleasant flavour and high "shortening" power. Such a fat creams easily and makes a light cake or pudding mixture or a short pastry. Lard, cooking fats and oils have a high shortening power and make the shortest pastry. Butter and margarine are most suitable for cakes because of their superior flavour.

For frying purposes, a fat should be free from moisture that would make it splutter when heated. If fats are heated beyond a certain temperature they begin to decompose into fatty acids and glycerol, give off blue acrolein smoke and this is the hazing point. If heating is continued decomposition increases, and there is a high risk of fire.

The solid fats and olive oil traditionally used for frying "haze" at comparatively low temperatures; so they are heated to the point where they begin to haze and then the food is put in for frying. The modern cooking oils have higher hazing temperatures and if one waits till they haze before starting to fry the food will cook too quickly and burn on the outside. To find the correct temperature one must either use a sample of food for testing, or a special thermometer. A fat with too low a hazing temperature cannot be used for frying satisfactorily as the food will cook too slowly and will not "seal" on the outside so that the fat will penetrate right into it.

Increasing use is now being made of vegetable oils for frying as well as for pastry-making, cakes, puddings and salad creams, dressings and mayonnaise. The most important of these vegetable oils are olive oil, corn oil or maize oil, and sunflower seed oil. The smoking point of cooking oils is higher than that of most cooking fats, and, since they are free from water, there is no spluttering during frying. Their being liquids makes it easier to gauge the amount required, since it covers the surface of the pan to the right depth immediately. In addition, the use of vegetable cooking oils helps to ensure a correct balance between animal and vegetable fat intake, which is important to health.

SUGAR

The chemical nature and food value of the different sugars have already been described in Chapter 2. The sugar we are concerned with here is the ordinary sugar we buy from the grocer. This is the sucrose derived from either sugar cane or sugar beet.

Sucrose is obtained from sugar canes by crushing them and then extracting with water. By heating, adding lime and bubbling carbon dioxide through the liquid, various impurities separate out and are skimmed off. The remaining liquid is then evaporated until concentrated enough to crystallise. The crystals are impure *brown sugar* and the liquid left is *molasses or treacle*.

Brown sugar is refined by dissolving it in water, filtering through bone charcoal and bleaching the solution with sulphur dioxide. The liquid is then concentrated in special vacuum pans until it crystallises. The crystals are now pure *white sugar* and the liquid left is *golden syrup*.

Sucrose is obtained from sugar beet in a very similar manner but the molasses from sugar beet is too impure to be used as human food.

The refined sugars from sugar cane and sugar beet are identical. They consist of approximately 99·5% pure sucrose and are exactly alike in appearance and sweetness.

Cane sugar has been known for more than two thousand years and has been used in this country for over six hundred years. Beet sugar has only been in use since the middle of the last century. As will be seen from the map the sugar cane grows in countries with a tropical or sub-tropical climate while sugar beet grows in countries with a temperate climate. Sugar beet is grown in this country.

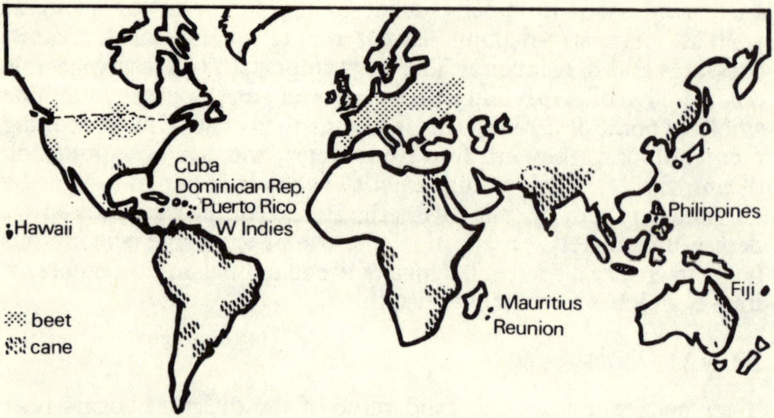

Sugar-producing areas of the world.

FORMS OF SUGAR

The most important processed forms of sugar in general use are granulated, cube or lump, castor, icing and demerara. *Granulated sugar* is in the form of small cubic crystals and is the commonest form of all. *Cube or lump sugar* is granulated sugar that has been caked into a hard mass and then cut into cubes by machinery. *Castor and icing sugars* are prepared from granulated sugar by milling to a fine powder and then sifting through silk sieves. The particles too big to pass through the silk form castor sugar: those fine enough to pass through form the icing sugar. *Demerara sugar* is an unrefined brown sugar.

SUGAR DERIVATIVES

Sugar Candy

This is prepared by suspending thin strings in a hot concentrated sugar solution. The sugar slowly crystallises on the strings in the form of large cubic crystals.

Barley Sugar

When sugar is heated it melts at about 101–104°C. If a little water is previously added it melts at a slightly lower temperature. The melted sugar becomes straw-coloured and, if allowed to cool at this stage, sets to a hard brittle mass of barley sugar. When prepared by confectioners it is either poured into moulds or on to a greased slab and, while still fairly plastic, cut with a sharp knife into strips which are then twisted between the finger and thumb.

Caramel

On further heating, sugar darkens in colour and, at about 176° C, is converted into a dark brown substance known as caramel. This has the smell and taste of burnt sugar and is much used as a colouring and flavouring in gravy browning, sauces, "artificial" vinegar, rich cakes, beer and stout.

Fondants

Fondants are really of two types—those used by sugar boilers as sweets and those used by confectioners for cake decorations. The principles underlying their preparation are, however, the same in both cases and consist in the formation of a sugar syrup which sets hard on cooling without crystallising. In other words, it sets hard without going sugary or crumbly as does an ordinary sugar syrup. This "cutting of the grain," as it is called, is accomplished either by adding some glucose to the cane sugar or converting some of the cane sugar (sucrose) into glucose and fructose by heating it with an acid substance, e.g., cream of tartar, tartaric or citric acid or vinegar. The presence of even a small amount of glucose in a cane sugar syrup prevents the sugar from crystallising, i.e., going crumbly, on cooling or keeping. The conversion of the double sugar, sucrose, into the single sugars, glucose and fructose, is known as "inversion." The cane sugar is said to be "inverted" and the mixture of glucose and fructose is known as "invert sugar."

It will be found that all fondant and toffee recipes include either glucose itself, or treacle or golden syrup, both of which contain glucose, or, alternatively, small amounts of such acid substances as cream of tartar, tartaric acid, lemon juice, acetic acid or vinegar are included. During the boiling of sugar syrup the acid substance inverts sufficient cane sugar to glucose to prevent crystallisation and the fondant or toffee sets hard. The same kind of inversion takes place in jam making due to the acid of the fruit.

The preparation of fondant can be illustrated in the following way. Heat 900 g of sugar with just over 0·25 litre of water in a copper or enamelled saucepan and add either 110 g glucose or a little cream of tartar, tartaric acid, lemon juice, acetic acid or vinegar.

Gradually raise the temperature to 118° C (soft ball degree on a sugar boiler's thermometer). Pour the syrup into a glazed earthenware basin and allow to cool to about 38° C. Stir the syrup with a wooden spoon. The syrup becomes more and more viscous and also less transparent and more creamy in appearance. When the sugar becomes too stiff to be stirred with the spoon, knead it with the hands until a smooth creamy mass is obtained. This is fondant such as is used for icing cakes and in sweetmeats.

If the sugar syrup had been poured out on to a greased slab and while still hot and plastic had been held in the two hands and thrown over a hook in the wall and pulled and twisted a number of times it would have gone fibrous and shiny and set to "rock." This pulling and folding, for which confectioners use a special machine, causes a partial crystallisation of the sugar but the crystals are too small to cause the rock to go sugary and crumbly.

Toffees and Sweets

We have seen that when sugar is heated it first of all melts and on continued heating turns dark brown to caramel. On still further heating it turns black to form sugar charcoal or carbon and finally burns completely away. In actual fact there are a large number of gradual changes in the sugar between melting and caramelisation which are not easy to distinguish except by the experienced eye. An expert sugar boiler can recognise ten different and distinct stages or "degrees" as follows:

Syrup	102–104° C
"Thread" degree	107° C
"Pearl" degree	110° C
"Blow" degree	113° C
"Feather" degree	116° C
"Soft ball" degree	118° C
"Hard ball" degree	121° C
"Soft crack" degree	138° C
"Hard crack" degree	155° C
Caramel	178° C

These various "degrees" can be determined best by the use of a sugar boiler's thermometer on which they are marked or, in skilled hands, by the shape and consistency of a sample of the syrup poured into water. For ordinary purposes only four of these degrees are of any real importance. They are:

107° C Thread degree for boiled icing.
118° C Soft ball degree for fondants.
155° C Crack degree for toffee.
178° C for colouring and flavouring.

If a thermometer is not available the following tests can be used:

Thread Degree

A little of the syrup is dropped from a wooden spoon into cold water. A thread is formed when the syrup is squeezed between finger and thumb and then separated.

Soft Ball Degree

A sample is dropped into cold water from a wooden spoon and when worked between the finger and thumb forms a soft ball.

Crack Degree

At this stage a sample poured into cold water will crackle and when taken out will be hard and brittle.

Caramel

The sugar begins to darken rapidly in colour and the smell of burnt sugar becomes noticeable.

The preparation of toffee can be illustrated in the following way. Place 55 g butter; 220 g treacle; 220 g cane sugar and a little lemon juice or vinegar in a clean saucepan. Bring to a boil and continue boiling until "crack" degree is reached. (Use a sugar boiler's thermometer or pour a sample into cold water.) Pour into a greased tin and stand in a cool place until set.

The butter in the recipe provides flavour and increases the food value, the treacle supplies glucose and the lemon juice or vinegar "inverts" some of the cane sugar during the boiling and so "cuts the grain." Such a toffee sets hard and does not go crumbly on keeping. The tin into which the toffee is poured is greased so that there will be a film of oil between the hot syrup and the tin. This prevents the toffee from sticking to the tin and it is easily removed.

HONEY

Honey is deposited by bees in the cells of wax combs and is obtained by them from the nectar of flowers. The sugar of nectar is cane sugar (sucrose) but as it passes through the bodies of the bees it is "inverted" and honey consists of about 75% of invert sugar (glucose and fructose). The flavour and aroma of honey are due to the scents derived from the flowers the bees have visited. The two main flavours are those of heather and clover.

Genuine honey is sometimes blended with artificial invert sugar but the fact must be stated on the label for such a mixture cannot legally be described as honey.

Honey is a very attractive and palatable energy food. During ancient and mediaeval times it was the chief source of sweetening materials. It was also fermented into a drink known as mead.

TREACLE AND GOLDEN SYRUP

We have already seen that these are by-products of the manufacture of granulated sugar. They remain syrups because of the invert sugar (glucose and fructose) which they contain in addition to cane sugar. Treacle contains, in addition to sugars, useful amounts of calcium and iron, but little is normally eaten.

CHOCOLATE

Chocolate is made from ground cocoa nibs, cocoa butter, cane sugar and flavourings. Milk chocolate has milk powder added to it. Chocolate is an acceptable energy food because of its sugar and fat. It contains useful amounts of iron derived from the cocoa nibs. Milk chocolate, because of its milk, contains valuable calcium and vitamins A, B and D.

Jams and dried fruits, which are usually classed as energy foods, are discussed in the chapter on the preservation of foods. (See Chapter 15.)

9 Fruits, Vegetables, Pulses and Nuts

FRUITS

To the botanist a fruit is the complete structure formed by the ovary of a flower after its ovules have been fertilised by pollen. It contains the seeds which must be dispersed if the life cycle is to be completed. Various methods of dispersal are adoped by different plants. Some seeds are dispersed by wind, some by water and others by mechanical means. Many plants envelop their seeds with succulent pulpy flesh with an attractive flavour and conspicuous colour. Birds, animals and human beings are tempted to eat these fruits and the hard, indigestible seeds they contain are liberated and dispersed. It is these succulent fruits which we call, in common parlance, "fruits." To the botanist, the dandelion "clock," the coconut, the pea pod, thistle "down" and the rose hip are just as much fruits as are the orange, tomato, apple or plum. Apples, apricots, bananas, blackberries, cherries, black, red and white currants, plums, damsons, greengages, lemons, loganberries, melons, oranges, peaches, pears, pineapples, raspberries, strawberries and tangerines are examples of succulent fruits. The tomato is a succulent fruit which is usually eaten as a vegetable. Rhubarb is eaten as a fruit but is, of course, a leaf stalk.

The general composition of ripe fresh fruit is approximately:

Water	85–90%
Protein	0·5%
Fat	0·5%
Carbohydrate	5·5–10·5%
Cellulose	2·5%
Minerals	0·5%

It will be seen from this table that we eat fruit more for its sweetness and flavour than for actual nourishment. There is always a very considerable amount of waste and a very large amount of water. The quantities of protein and fat are so small as to be

G

negligible. Olives and Avocado pears, which contain a large proportion of fat, are exceptions. In unripe fruits the carbohydrate is mainly starch but as the fruits ripen the enzymes and acids they contain gradually change the starch into sucrose (cane sugar) and the sucrose into fructose and glucose. The "unavailable" carbohydrates consist chiefly of cellulose and pectin and are of no food value since they are indigestible. The cellulose serves a useful purpose in acting as roughage and the pectin is important in helping the fruit to set to a jelly in jam-making. The amounts of cellulose and pectin vary greatly in different fruits. They are always less in cultivated fruits than in the corresponding wild fruits, e.g., crab apples contain much more than cultivated apples. The amounts also diminish during the ripening of fruit.

The minerals in fruit are chiefly the potassium salts of various "fruit acids"—tartaric, citric and malic acids. These give fruits their agreeable acid flavours. During ripening the amounts of these acids diminish while the amounts of sugar increase. This alteration in the balance of sour acid and sweet sugar flavourings accounts for the difference in taste between unripe and ripe fruits. Fruit acids are also necessary, along with sugar, to cause pectin to set to a jelly in jam making. Reasonable amounts of iron are found in a few fruits e.g., black and red currants, loganberries, but the small amounts we normally eat do not add a significant amount to the diet.

The large amounts of indigestible cellulose in fruits by providing roughage has a useful laxative action.

Fresh fruits, with the exceptions of apples, pears, plums and cherries, are important sources of ascorbic acid, while the yellow fruits, apricots, peaches and oranges, contain some carotene and so do tomatoes. In the case of tomatoes the yellow colour of the carotene is masked by a red pigment. In spite of its lack of ascorbic acid, the apple is a valuable fruit. Its hardness helps to teach children to chew and cleans their teeth after meals.

The smell and flavour of fruits are due to the presence of very small quantities of essential oils, esters and ethers. Like the extractives of meat they have no food value in themselves but stimulate the appetite and so promote digestion.

It will thus be seen that from the nutritional angle fresh fruits are mainly valuable for their ascorbic acid content. They are protective foods and the most valuable fruits are those which contain most ascorbic acid. These, as we have previously seen, are *the summer fruits*, blackcurrants, gooseberries, strawberries, raspberries and tomatoes and *the imported citrus fruits*, oranges, lemons and grapefruits. Because of the fact that they can be eaten practically all the year round tomatoes and oranges are especially valuable. The other fruits not mentioned are not so valuable as green vegetables as sources of ascorbic acid and are mainly to be regarded as providing pleasant taste, attractiveness to meals and variety in the diet. Because of the destructive action of heat upon ascorbic acid fruit should preferably be eaten raw. The acidity of the fruit and its skin both help to preserve the ascorbic acid during storage. Care should be taken not to bruise or damage fruit since ascorbic acid is destroyed when the cells containing it are ruptured and their enzymes liberated to attack the vitamin.

Fruit drinks are refreshing and when made from fresh fruit rich in ascorbic acid, e.g., lemons, oranges and blackcurrants, can be a good source of this vitamin. Blackcurrant juice, rose hip syrup and concentrated orange juice are extremely valuable sources of ascorbic acid and consequently are strongly recommended for young children, but they should be suitably diluted. The blackcurrant cordials and rose hip syrup have a lot of sugar added to them and are as dangerous as sweets are to a child's teeth.

Manufactured drinks such as mineral waters, lemonade and fruit cordials contain at most only a negligible amount of ascorbic acid.

VEGETABLES

A great variety of plants and of different parts of them are eaten as vegetables. A rough classification of the vegetables used in this country is as follows:

(1) *Green leaves*
Lettuce, watercress, cabbage, sprouts, spinach, broccoli, mustard and cress, turnip tops, kale, savoys, parsley.

(2) *Inflorescences (Flower buds)*
Cauliflower, broccoli.

(3) *Leaf stalks*
Celery and rhubarb.

(4) *Stems*
Asparagus, sea-kale.

(5) *Roots*
Carrot, parsnip, beetroot, swede, turnip, radish.

(6) *Tubers*
Potato, Jerusalem artichoke.

(7) *Bulbs*
Onion, leek, garlic.

(8) *Fruits and Seeds*
Cucumber, marrow, tomato, pulses (peas, beans), mushrooms.

This long list can be grouped into two main types:
(*a*) The green leafy vegetables. (*b*) Bulbs, roots and tubers.

(1) Green Leafy Vegetables and **(2) Inflorescences**

The green vegetables are those whose leaves are used as food. The leaves of a plant act as the factories for the production of sugar which is then carried away to other parts of the plant either to be used at once or stored as starch for future use.

The thin layer of the leaf in between the upper and lower skins consists, for the most part, of living cells in which is contained the green chlorophyll enclosed in compartments of cellulose. Chlorophyll has the power of abstracting energy from sunlight which the living stuff of the cells (protoplasm) uses to convert carbon dioxide obtained from the air and water from the soil into sugar. Vitamins, minerals and enzymes are agents in bringing about this chemical change and are particularly abundant and active in leaves.

The inflorescences are the flowers of the vegetable.

The leaves and flowers are not storage organs and consequently contain very little protein, fat or carbohydrate. Their value in the diet depends upon the vitamins and minerals they contain. Like fresh fruits they are neither body-building nor energy foods. They provide little in the way of amino-acids or energy, but they are valuable protective foods.

The most important minerals in vegetables are calcium and iron. Unlike the other minerals present—sodium, potassium, magnesium, phosphorus and chlorine—they are not dissolved out when green vegetables are cooked but the amounts in an average helping are not large and, as previously mentioned, are not always fully "available."

It is chiefly as sources of vitamins that these vegetables are of such importance in the diet. They are all, except cauliflowers and broccoli, rich sources of carotene from which the body can make vitamin A. The greener and leafier the vegetable the greater is the amount of carotene. Thus the outside leaves of cabbage and lettuce, which are often discarded, contain more carotene than the white hearts. In the fresh raw state, most of the leafy and flowering vegetables are rich sources of ascorbic acid, and this is their greatest merit. It has already been emphasised that a loss of ascorbic acid occurs when green vegetables are stored, especially if bruised or damaged, and a further loss when cooked. For this reason they should always be eaten as fresh as possible. Raw salads are a good source of ascorbic acid and can be eaten all the year round, for a good salad is not merely a lot of lettuce leaves with a few radishes, but a mixture of all kinds of raw vegetables in season. Thus with a little ingenuity it is possible to devise an attractive and nutritious salad at any time of the year.

Suitable ingredients for salads include:

Green leafy vegetables such as cabbage, savoy, sprouts, spinach, young kale and young turnip tops, watercress, lettuce and endive.
Root vegetables such as raw or cooked beetroot, turnip, carrot, swede and parsnip.
Other vegetables such as cooked potatoes, raw radishes, cucumber, leeks, onions, cooked or raw peas, cooked french or runner beans, celery, cauliflower, broccoli and cooked broad beans.
Flavourings such as green herbs, chives, mint, parsley, spring onions, young celery leaves, nasturtium and dandelion leaves, mustard and cress.
Fruit of any kind, fresh or dried.
Eggs, either fresh or dried, served scrambled or hardboiled.
Cheese either grated or cut in cubes or slices.
Meat and fish, cooked or canned.

Such salads can be served as a small helping with hot meat, fish or other savoury dish, or as a filling for sandwiches or rolls. Alternatively, the salad could be served as the main dish of a meal with meat, fish, cheese or eggs and bread or potatoes; as a substitute for the sweet course or at the beginning of a meal in place of soup. For those who like it a creamy salad dressing adds to the flavour and supplies fat.

Green leafy vegetables are not particularly good sources of the B group of vitamins. There is little likelihood of destruction of vitamin B_1 (thiamine) at the temperatures used in cooking unless bicarbonate of soda is added to preserve the green colour of the vegetables. A good deal, however, passes into the cooking water since the thiamine is very soluble.

(3) Leafy stalks

Rhubarb which is a leafy stalk and therefore really a vegetable is normally regarded as a fruit. It has a useful vitamin C content but contains a lot of oxalic acid which renders its calcium insoluble and therefore unavailable.

Celery which used to be regarded as a seasonal vegetable is now available all year round. It contains some calcium.

(4) Stems

The main nutritive value of these is in the sauces served with them, but they do also contain vitamin C.

(5) Bulbs (6) Roots (7) Tubers

Unlike the green leafy parts of vegetables, bulbs, roots and tubers are storage organs in which the sugars and starch manufactured by the leaves are collected for future use by the plant. The roots, bulbs and tubers we eat are those of plants which require two years for complete growth. They are biennials which spend the first season of growth storing up food for use in their second season when they form their flowers and seeds. When cultivated for food they are, of course, only grown for one reason, i.e., they are grown as annuals.

Roots, tubers and bulbs are thus quite distinct from green leafy vegetables and serve a different purpose in the diet. In spite of the large amounts of water and cellulose they contain, many of them are valuable energy foods because of their starch and sugar and some contain a small amount of valuable protein, minerals and vitamins.

The potato is a tuber and is the most valuable of this type of vegetable. After the cereals, it is, in fact, the most important plant food. It contains a comparatively large amount of starch so that it is a good source of energy, and a small amount of protein especially just below the skin. It is not rich in mineral salts but it has valuable amounts of ascorbic acid, some thiamine, and a little carotene. The fact that there is a loss of ascorbic acid when potatoes are stored and a further loss when cooked, particularly when mashed or kept hot for long periods after cooking, has previously been stated. All the same, potatoes are eaten so regularly and in such large amounts compared with other vegetables that they make an important contribution to our supplies of ascorbic acid. Potatoes have the further merit of a very mild flavour so that we do not quickly tire of them and they form an admirable medium for mixing with a great variety of other foodstuffs such as milk, meat, fish and eggs.

The roots, such as carrot, swede, parsnip and beetroot, contain more water and less starch than the potato and have, consequently, less energy value. They contain varying amounts of ascorbic acid, swedes and turnips being the richest sources among the root vegetables. They have little of the B group of vitamins and, with the notable exception of the carrot, very little carotene.

The chief bulb vegetable is *the onion* which is especially rich in sugar. The essential oil the onion contains gives it its pungency which is so useful in the flavouring of many otherwise insipid dishes.

(8) Fruits and Seeds

Green peas and broad beans contain more carbohydrate and protein than other vegetables. They also contain some ascorbic acid and, in the case of green peas, carotene as well. *French and runner beans* are useful for both carotene and ascorbic acid.

Tomatoes contain valuable amounts of ascorbic acid and carotene. Tinned tomatoes and tomato juice and purée contain the vitamins though in reduced amounts.

Other vegetables such as *cucumber* and *marrow* contain so little nutriment that they can only be regarded as pleasant adjuncts to the diet.

The *edible fungi*—mushrooms and truffles—are of little importance in the diet. Their food value is negligible and they are difficult to digest. Their flavour is their only recommendation. They are condiments rather than foods.

In the case of all vegetables as in the case of fruits and the husks of cereals, the indigestible cellulose of the vegetables increases the bulk of the diet, acts as roughage and stimulates the peristaltic action of the intestines which is so frequently necessary in the highly concentrated and refined diets so commonly taken today.

Finally, the vegetables add flavour and variety to the diet and form an excellent medium for the addition of other nutrients, e.g., the fat and milk used in the sauces frequently served with them.

The preservation of fruits and vegetables is discussed in Chapter 15, and their cooking in Chapter 16.

PULSES

By the term pulses we usually mean dried peas, beans and lentils which are the seeds formed in the pods or shells of leguminous plants, but the term can conveniently be extended to include the seeds of other leguminous plants used as human food such as the soya bean and the peanut (monkey nut or groundnut). You will remember that leguminous plants are those which are able, with the help of bacteria in nodules on their roots, to form their protein from the nitrogen of the air. One of the characteristics of the pulses is the relatively large amount of protein they contain, which can be valuable when used as a supplement to the protein of meat, fish and eggs. This is their chief value. They are a cheap protein supplement. It should be realised, however, that the protein of pulses, legumin, is inferior to that of the cereals and that, in this country, pulses are not normally eaten in large amounts except by vegetarians.

In addition to their protein, dry pulses in general have a high starch and sugar content and consequently a high energy value. They are rich in calcium, phosphorus, iron and vitamins of the B group. Peas, beans and lentils are deficient in fat and it is a good plan to serve them along with fatty protein foods such as pork and bacon.

Dried pulses need to be soaked before cooking. It is best to cover them with boiling water and soak overnight. The boiling precipitates calcium carbonate from hard water which would otherwise be absorbed by the pulses and contribute to their hardening. If the water is very hard, or the pulses very old and hard, bicarbonate of soda may be used to soften the water and the tissues of the pulses. During the soaking the pulses take up a considerable amount of water with consequent increase in weight and bulk. This makes their food value *as eaten* much less than might be supposed from an examination of food tables showing the composition of dried pulses.

Besides long soaking, pulses also need long cooking unless finely divided as in pea flour, otherwise they are apt to be indigestible and cause flatulence. Probably most of the vitamin B_1 (thiamine) of the pulses is lost or destroyed during the soaking and cooking with bicarbonate of soda so that they lose any protective value they might possess. It is doubtful if much of the iron they contain is "available." There is no ascorbic acid in dried pulses but it can be developed in them by steeping them in cold water and allowing them to stand until germination begins. This method is excellent with dried peas. The amount of carotene in dried pulses is negligible.

The soya bean is a native of Eastern Asia and one of the oldest crops grown by man. It has probably been cultivated in China for more than five thousand years. In China, Japan and neighbouring countries the soya bean is one of the most important articles of diet. For the poorer classes it forms one of the principal sources of protein. It is described as "the meat without bones." The beans can be picked green and cooked or served raw in salads or the dried beans can be soaked in salt water and then roasted. A vegetable milk is made from the crushed beans as a substitute for animal milk.

In recent years its use has spread to other countries and attempts have been made to cultivate it in many parts of the world. The soya bean has been successfully grown in America and is used in breakfast foods, beverages and soup powders; the oil crushed from the beans is used in margarine, cooking oils and salad oils. In this country its cultivation has not yet proved successful but increasing amounts are imported for the preparation of soya bean flour which is used in soups, meat loaves, gravies, sauces, stews, pastes, sandwich spreads, biscuits, puddings and custards.

Soya flour does not thicken when cooked as do wheat flour and cornflour because of the smaller amount of carbohydrate it contains. Consequently, for thickening sauces, stews and gravies it can only be used in combination with wheat flour or cornflour. Since it contains a large proportion of fat and no gluten it cannot be used alone in making cakes, biscuits or pastry. They would be too heavy to be palatable. Soya flour does not bind well and will not rise. By using soya flour in the proportion of one part of soya to seven parts of wheat flour excellent bread, cakes, biscuits, pastry and so on can be made and their food value enhanced. Soya flour is sold in this country in a form suitable for making milk puddings. It could be more extensively used with advantage.

The soya bean differs from peas, beans and lentils in having a large proportion of fat and, therefore, a much higher energy value.

It also contains rather more protein, of a higher biological value and more of the B group of vitamins and more calcium and iron. The amount of carbohydrate is correspondingly less.

NUTS

Nuts are highly nutritious foods because of their protein, fat and mineral salts. They have, however, a large proportion of waste and owing to their fat and the tough fibrous framework of cellulose are rather indigestible. For this reason, nuts should always be well chewed, minced or crushed to flour. Alternatively, they can be cooked before eating. Almonds and walnuts contain vitamin B_1 (thiamine). With the exception of the chestnut the amounts of carbohydrates are low. The chestnut contains much less fat than other nuts.

The protein of nuts is of low biological value but it is supplemented by the protein of milk, cheese and eggs. The calcium and iron of nuts is probably not all "available" because of the presence of phytic acid. The fat of nuts is quite exceptional in amount for vegetable foods and gives them a high energy value. These vegetable fats are lacking in vitamins A and D but are used in very large quantities in the preparation of margarine.

Non vegetarians use nuts merely as a dessert and they play only a small part in their diet, mainly because of their high cost.

The peanut, earthnut, groundnut or monkey nut is strictly speaking a fruit (and not a nut) as it grows on an annual plant. The fruit matures in the ground and the kernel grows inside pods like peas—hence its alternative names.

However, since it is always thought of as a nut it is considered under this heading.

The peanut has a high protein and fat content. The protein is not of a high biological value as some of the essential amino-acids are missing. The fat, which amounts to more than 40%, is crushed out of the peanuts and used very extensively in the preparation of margarine, cooking fat and the peanut butter used by vegetarians.

10 Milk

Milk is the creamy yellow liquid formed by all female mammals for feeding their young. Cows' milk is the one most commonly used in this country but the milks of ewes, goats, mares, asses and reindeer are used as human food in various parts of the world. The milks of different animals are very similar to one another and contain the same food materials but with slight differences in composition and in proportions.

Milk is often spoken of as "Nature's most perfect food." This expression may, perhaps, give an exaggerated idea of its qualities but it is true to say that milk is the most complete single food we know. Since cows' milk is the only food of the young calf, it must necessarily contain all the food ingredients needed for its life and growth. While not a complete food for human beings, cows' milk is, nevertheless, of the very greatest value at all stages of human life and particularly to children, adolescents, expectant and nursing mothers, invalids and old people.

Milk contains every type of nutrient, i.e., carbohydrate, fat, protein, minerals and vitamins. Its proteins are animal proteins of high biological value. It is exceptionally rich in calcium and phosphorus, and has a generous supply of vitamin A and riboflavin along with useful amounts of the other members of the vitamin B complex. Cows' milk contains ascorbic acid, vitamin D and iron but not in sufficient amounts even for a young child. As previously mentioned, infants fed entirely on cows' milk need additional amounts of ascorbic acid and vitamin D and, after six months of age, additional iron in order to obtain a complete diet.

A ½ litre milk supplies a child of five years with all the calcium, riboflavin and vitamin A, nearly half the protein and a third of the thiamine required daily. For an average man a ½ litre milk supplies all the calcium and vitamin A, a quarter of the protein, nearly half the riboflavin and one sixth of the thiamine. In view of these remarkable facts it is not surprising that a bottle of milk is so often recommended as the basis of our daily diet, that additional milk is provided for some children at school, and that toddlers and expectant and nursing mothers are given priority in milk supplies during times of scarcity.

The exact composition of milk varies somewhat with the particular breed of cow, the length of time since it had a calf, the nature of the food it has eaten and the season of the year. The variations in the amounts of protein, calcium and phosphorus are not large, but the amounts of vitamin A vary considerably with the cow's food, the amounts of vitamin D with the season, and the amounts of ascorbic acid with the state of the milk, i.e., whether it is raw, pasteurised, sterilised, or boiled, and whether or not it has been left exposed to light. The following composition is an average one based on thousands of analyses.

Water	87·54%
Protein	3·29%
Fat	3·71%
Carbohydrate ..	4·70%
Minerals	0·76%
	100·00%

Total Solids = 12·46%.
Total Solids (not fat) = 8·75%.

MILK PROTEINS

The chief protein in milk is known as *caseinogen*. It is a very valuable body-building material containing phosphorus which is needed for the nervous tissues. With it are smaller amounts of two other proteins known as *lactalbumen* and *lactoglobulin*. Caseinogen is similar to the vitellin of egg yolk, while lactalbumen and lactoglobulin are similar to the proteins of white of egg.

When milk is turned sour by bacteria on keeping, its sugar, lactose, is converted into lactic acid and the milk becomes so acid that the caseinogen is rendered insoluble in the water of the milk and is precipitated as a curd. We say the milk has curdled. Other acids such as vinegar, lemon juice, cream of tartar and tartaric acid produce a similar effect.

In the stomachs of babies and small children there is a substance called *rennin* (see p. 286) which changes the caseinogen of milk to casein, and this combines with the calcium of the milk to form an insoluble mass or *clot*. This clot shrinks, becomes entangled with the fat of the milk, thus forming a curd and subsequently expresses a yellowish liquid called whey. There is thus a distinction between the acid curdling and rennin clotting of milk. An extract of rennin, known as *rennet*, which is obtained from a calf's stomach, can be bought from the chemist's. It is used to make milk into junket and cheese. When rennet is used the milk has to be warmed to blood-heat, 36·9° C, since this is the temperature at which rennin is accustomed to working in our stomachs and those of calves.

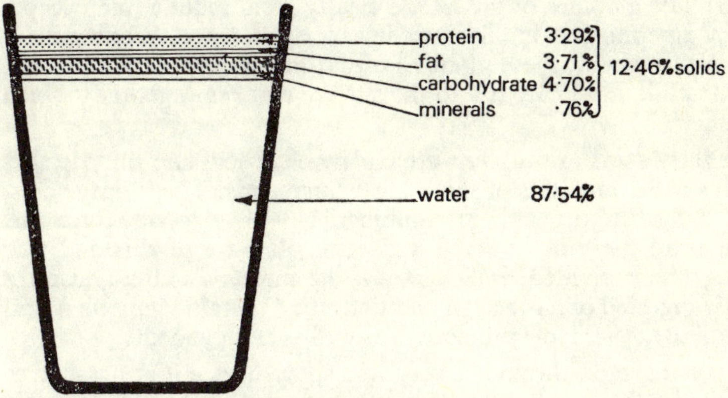

Percentage composition of milk.

When milk is poured into a strong infusion of tea, it is clotted by the tannin, the harsh taste of which is consequently reduced. Hence the use of milk in tea.

The lactalbumen and lactoglobulin of milk are not curdled by bacteria or acids or clotted by rennet but when milk is heated they set (coagulate) and form a skin on the surface at about 71° C. It is the collection of air bubbles and steam under this skin which causes milk to boil over so easily when it is heated above this temperature. Caseinogen does not ordinarily coagulate with heat unless the milk is nearly sour.

All three proteins of milk are animal proteins of the highest biological value. As we would expect, they contain all the essential amino-acids, in a proper balance, and are extremely valuable body-building materials. In addition, they have the further merit of being easily digested and of greatly increasing the value of any plant proteins eaten along with them at the same meal. This supplementing of plant proteins occurs when milk is used with flour in making bread, scones, teacakes, buns and cakes, and with cereals such as oatmeal in porridge and rice in puddings.

MILK FATS

The fat of fresh milk is in the form of tiny globules dispersed throughout the water of the milk. Such a mixture of fat and water is called an emulsion. (Fat and water do not, of course, ordinarily mix.) The globules of fat can be clearly seen under a microscope. They give milk its "milky" opalescent appearance. When milk is allowed to stand, these globules of fat, being lighter than the rest of the milk, gradually rise to the surface and run together to form cream.

The fatty acids in milk fats are chiefly oleic acid and butyric acid with smaller amounts of some other fatty acids. These fatty acids, especially butyric acid, in combination with glycerin, form fats which are pleasant in smell and taste. Because of this and also being finely divided, milk fats are the most palatable and most easily digested of all fats. In addition, they contain vitamins A and D and so are valuable protectives as well as energy foods.

By passing milk through a very fine spray nozzle it is possible to break the fat droplets up even further so that the fat is evenly dispersed throughout the milk and will not rise up to the surface as cream. This process of breaking up the droplets is called *homogenisation.*

MILK SUGAR

Milk sugar or lactose is a double sugar, i.e., disaccharide. It is the only carbohydrate in milk and is the only known animal sugar. It has very little sweetness compared with cane sugar. This is probably an advantage since we would tire quickly of milk if it had a strong taste. There is no difference in their energy values.

The bacteria which turn milk sour are known as lactic acid bacteria. They feed upon the lactose of milk and change it into lactic acid which curdles the caseinogen. The milk goes sour and separates into curds and whey.

Cows' milk contains more protein than human milk and infants find difficulty in digesting it. Therefore, cows' milk has to be diluted and some carbohydrate added to restore its energy value per gramme. This is usually lactose (natural milk sugar) which is preferable to the sucrose (cane sugar) formerly used. Milk puddings, in which a large proportion of starchy carbohydrate, e.g., rice, sago, tapioca, is added to milk and sweetened with sugar, make a more correctly balanced food for children and adults. Custards, made with starchy custard powder and milk, or milk and biscuits, serve the same purpose.

MILK MINERALS

Milk contains all the minerals necessary for the growth of the young animal. The important ones are calcium and phosphorus, which are essential for the formation of sound bones and teeth. Milk is the best source of these two food minerals.

It has already been emphasised that milk is deficient in iron so that young infants fed on milk require additional iron after six months of age if they are not to become anaemic. This is usually supplied by the egg yolk, finely minced liver or sieved green vegetables that are given to babies as they go on to a more solid diet.

MILK VITAMINS

All the commoner vitamins are present in milk in varying amounts. Vitamin A is present in considerable amounts in the milk fats. The actual amount depends largely on the cow's food and is greater in summer when the cows graze on quickly growing herbage than in winter when they are fed on hay and other winter fodder. Vitamin D is also present in the milk fats but the amount is small and variable. Like vitamin A it is greatest in milk during the summer when the cows are out in the sunshine and in the field. Babies fed on cows' milk need additional supplies of vitamins A and D from halibut liver oil or cod liver oil or vitamin drops.

Milk is a good source of riboflavin throughout the year although some of it is destroyed if the milk is left exposed to ordinary daylight or, still more, to bright sunlight. Thiamine and nicotinic acid are present in small amounts; the variation in amounts between summer and winter milk is but slight.

Milk is also a good source of the amino-acid tryptophane which the body can convert into the vitamin nicotinic acid.

Ascorbic acid is found in milk in small amounts only but this is remarkably constant as the milk leaves the cow. It is afterwards that the amount of ascorbic acid decreases according to the treatment the milk receives. Thus, a bottle of milk left on the doorstep in daylight or, worse still, direct sunlight, soon loses much of its ascorbic acid. The pasteurisation of milk causes some destruction of the vitamin and sterilisation, or boiling, is still more destructive. These facts emphasise the need of bottle-fed infants for the supplement of orange juice previously mentioned.

WATER OF MILK

Milk contains much more water than anything else. Seven-eighths of milk is water and only one-eighth solids. Of these solids, the fats are dispersed in the water as an emulsion and the rest are dissolved. By itself milk is thus a very dilute and bulky form of food for everybody except infants. It is apt to be regarded wrongly as a beverage instead of as a food.

BACTERIA IN MILK

Milk is not only a splendid food for animals and human beings but also, unfortunately, for bacteria. It contains all the essential nutrients, it is a liquid and it is handled a good deal. All these factors make milk particularly liable to infection by bacteria and for their rapid growth when once they have been introduced. Freshly drawn from a healthy and perfectly clean cow, milk is practically free from bacteria. On the other hand, milk from unhealthy cows is liable to contain disease bacteria. Tuberculosis and undulant fever can be passed on from cows to human beings in this way.

It is more common, however, for bacteria to be introduced into milk after it has been withdrawn. This is possible in a great many ways.

Dirty milk literally teems with bacteria. Dirt and bacteria may enter the milk from the cow's body, from dust and dirt in the cowshed, from the milker, from the milking apparatus and utensils, during transit to the consumer and in the home. The great majority of them are harmless to health and will do nothing worse to the milk than turn it sour, but serious outbreaks of scarlet fever, diphtheria, septic sore throat and typhoid have frequently been traced to milk infected by some carrier of these diseases.

A pure milk supply is of the very greatest importance to the health of the nation. There are two methods of tackling the problem. The first is to ensure that the cows in the dairy herd are perfectly healthy and are milked under conditions of perfect cleanliness, and that the milk is cooled and bottled as soon as possible. The second method is to destroy by heat any disease bacteria in milk, i.e., by sterilisation or pasteurisation. The first is the more ideal method but the second is the more practicable at the present time. The conviction is growing that even the purest milk should be pasteurised and that we should no more think of drinking raw milk than we would think of eating raw meat.

Sterilised Milk has been heated to not less than 100° C, for some time. This treatment destroys the bacteria but also alters the taste of the milk. The ascorbic acid is destroyed, the lactalbumen and lactoglobulin coagulated, and the fine emulsion of fat broken up. This type of milk has never become very popular but it keeps well.

The most usual method of sterilisation is to first homogenise the milk, then to bottle it and then to raise its temperature to 104° C for fifteen minutes, after which it is rapidly cooled.

However, now a new method of sterilising the milk can be used, this involves the use of a higher temperature, 132° C but for only 2 seconds. The shorter treatment time, though it sterilises the milk, has less effect on the taste.

Sterilising the milk alters its taste as it cooks some of the protein and burns the sugar. It also destroys all the vitamin C and much of the vitamin B_1, although the degree of damage will vary with the length of time the process takes. Consequently U.H.T. treatment is less damaging than the normal sterilising methods.

Pasteurised Milk (so called after Pasteur) has been heat treated to provide safe milk of good keeping quality without altering the taste or destroying the cream line as occurs with sterilisation.

The most usual method of pasteurisation requires that "the milk shall be maintained at a temperature of not less than 71·6° C, for at least fifteen seconds, and shall be immediately cooled to a temperature of not more than 11° C." Immediate cooling is required to ensure maximum effect from the treatment. Growth

H

of the surviving (all non-pathogenic) organisms is checked and keeping quality consequently further promoted. Such cooling is also important for the maximum restoration of the cream line.

As a result of pasteurisation the vitamin content of milk is altered to a varying degree. Vitamins A, riboflavin, D and E are not affected by pasteurisation. Vitamin B_1 may be reduced by 10 to 20%. Vitamin C is heat sensitive to a greater or less extent depending upon previous exposure to light, especially sunshine, and the degree of oxidation which has taken place. Usually the loss ranges from 20 to 40% of the vitamin C present in the raw milk prior to treatment. It should be realised that the quantity of vitamin C in raw milk is not large, certainly not sufficient to satisfy human requirements, and this deficiency must, in any case, be made good by foods other than milk.

FRESH MILK ON SALE

Farm-bottled milk. Milk that is not heat-treated and is bottled at the farm.
Pasteurised milk.
Homogenised pasteurised milk.
Sterilised milk.
Ultra-high temperature (U.H.T.) milk.

All milk on sale in this country is free from tuberculosis bacteria as all herds in this country are now free from this infection, but other disease-causing bacteria may be present in untreated milk. It is particularly important that children should be given heat-treated and not farm-bottled milk.

Treatment of Milk in the Home

It is no use buying clean milk unless it receives proper care in the home. The following points about the care of milk in the home are all too frequently overlooked:

(1) Never leave the milk on the doorstep exposed to sunlight.

(2) Keep in a cool dark place—in the refrigerator if you are fortunate enough to possess one.

(3) In hot weather stand the bottle in a basin of cold water with a piece of muslin over the top with the edges dipping in the water. If the basin can be stood in a draught so much the better. The muslin soaks up water which slowly evaporates. Heat is withdrawn

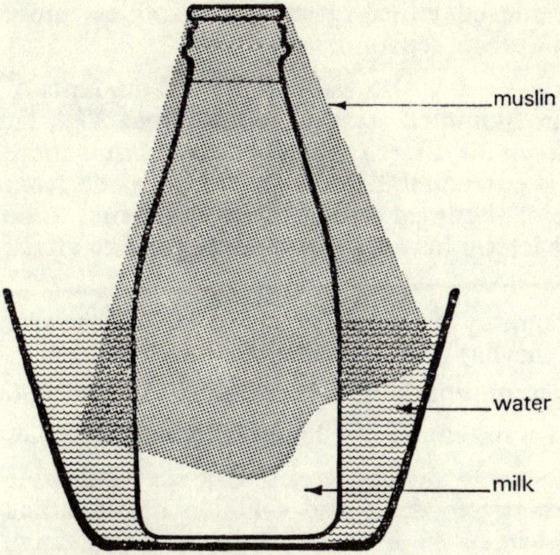

A simple milk-cooler.

from the milk to help this evaporation and the milk is thus kept cool.

(4) Do not pour the milk into jugs until required for use and see that the jugs are perfectly clean. Milk jugs should be washed in cold water, then in very hot water and finally rinsed in cold water. The jugs should be turned upside down to drain. The inside should not be dried with a teacloth. This may introduce bacteria.

(5) When milk is in the jug, keep it covered to protect it against dust and flies. Both may infect milk with bacteria.

(6) Never place milk near a sink or near foods with a strong smell, e.g., onions. The mild taste of milk is easily spoilt by the absorption of such smells.

(7) Never mix new milk with old milk unless it is to be used immediately; otherwise the bacteria in the old milk will quickly infect the new.

MILK PRODUCTS

Cream

We have seen that when milk is allowed to stand the fat globules rise to the surface and run together to form a layer of cream. This cream layer can be removed either by skimming off or, more efficiently, by means of a cream separator.

Cream contains not only fat but also water and small amounts of protein and milk sugar. Skimmed cream contains about 20% fat and separated cream about 50% fat. Separated cream is thus more concentrated. It also keeps better because it can be made from fresh milk. In the case of skimmed cream, the milk has first to be allowed to stand and bacteria have time to multiply and to attack the cream.

At one time it was customary to add preservatives and thickening materials to cream but this has been made illegal.

Single cream contains a minimum of 18% by weight of milk fat.

Double cream contains a minimum of 40% by weight of milk fat.

Because its fats are so finely divided cream is a very palatable and easily digested energy food. It also contains the vitamins A and D of the milk dissolved in it and is thus a protective food. It is a particularly suitable form of fat for invalids and convalescents.

Devonshire, Cornish or *clotted cream* is made by allowing milk to stand for twelve hours, then scalding it and allowing it to stand again before separating. Besides cream it contains most of the protein and sugar of the milk and resembles a very soft cream cheese.

Whipped cream can be best made from cream which is slightly sour. Fresh cream is not sufficiently acid for the emulsion of fat to break down easily during whipping. On the other hand, older cream, if too acid, is liable to whip to butter.

"*Reconstituted cream,*" which differs very little in appearance or taste from fresh cream, is made by emulsifying together salt-free butter and milk. Special machines are on sale for home use for this purpose.

"*Imitation cream,*" used for filling cakes and buns, is made by emulsifying together a mixture of unsalted butter or margarine, milk powder and water.

"*Ice cream,*" as sold in this country, is not frozen cream but a synthetic product made from milk powder, unsalted margarine, sugar and gelatine. Ice cream is an excellent food but the amounts usually eaten do not add much to the diet.

Butter

Butter is made by churning separated cream after it has "ripened." The ripening is a souring brought about by lactic acid bacteria. They form lactic acid which improves the flavour and breaks down the emulsion, thus helping the fat globules to stick together into a solid mass of butter. The solid lumps of butter are collected and moulded into shape after the addition of a little salt and colouring matter.

Butter contains about 85% fat. The rest is water with small amounts of salt and caseinogen. The presence of water and caseinogen favours the growth of bacteria which turn butter rancid. The salt helps to prevent this as well as giving flavour.

Butter is a very palatable and easily digested fat containing the vitamins A and D of the original milk. It is one of our most valuable energy foods. The volatile fats in butter, chiefly butyrin, give it its pleasant smell and taste. Its distinctive flavour is imparted to any cakes or other baked goods in which it is used.

Margarine

Margarine is not a milk product but it is convenient to discuss it here. It is made from a great variety of fats and oils such as beef fat, lard, olive, groundnut, cotton seed, palm kernel, sunflower and soya bean oils. Whale oils and fish oils and some vegetable oils, which were previously unsuitable for human food on account of their objectionable smell and taste, can now be refined and converted into palatable solid fats by a process of hydrogenation. This consists in passing hydrogen gas through them under special conditions. These hydrogenated fats and oils are now largely used in margarine and in cooking and frying fats.

The fats and oils are melted together so as to give a mixture with about the same melting point as butter and then emulsified with soured skim milk. The mixture is then rapidly frozen, allowed to mature for a short time and then kneaded to the correct consistency, salt and colouring matter being added.

Modern margarines contain about the same amount of fat as butter and have about the same kcal. value. The vitamins A and D which are absent from most of the fats and oils used in margarine are added to it during manufacture to make it equivalent in this respect to an average butter. Margarine does not contain the butyrin found in butter and thus lacks its pleasant smell and taste.

Some table margarines now have some butter added to improve their smell and taste, and some have a higher proportion of polyunsaturated fatty acids giving a 'soft' margarine. Some doctors claim these polyunsaturated fats are better for health than the more saturated fats.

Cheese

Cheese consists chiefly of the casein and fat of milk. It is prepared by souring the milk by the addition of an acid such as vinegar or by souring by bacteria. When the milk is sufficiently ripe, rennet is added to clot the protein. The whey is strained from the curd and the curd then salted and pressed to remove as much as possible of the remaining whey. Finally, it is set aside in a cool place to "ripen." The flavour and character of the cheese are developed during this stage by the action of bacteria and moulds.

The variations in taste, texture and appearance between different types of cheese are due to:

(1) *The type of milk used, e.g.*
Cheshire and Cheddar from whole cows' milk.
Stilton from milk to which additional cream has been added.
Parmesan from separated milk.
Gorgonzola from cows' and goats' milk.
Roquefort from ewes' milk.

(2) *The amount of pressing*
Hard cheeses such as Cheshire, Cheddar and Lancashire have been pressed in cheese presses.
Soft cheeses such as Stilton and Gorgonzola have been subjected only to the pressure of their own weight.

(3) *The amount and kind of ripening*
The particular flavour of a cheese depends upon the type of bacteria used in the ripening and the length of time it is allowed to proceed. Special green moulds are used in the ripening of such cheeses as Stilton and Gorgonzola.

"*Processed cheeses*" are made by grinding a mixture of cheeses to a fine powder, pasteurising then mixing them with water, salt and an emulsifier and then reheating, stirring the mixture so that a soft blended cheese is produced. The hot mixture is then poured into lined moulds.

Cheese spreads are made by adding whey, dried skimmed milk and sometimes cream, water and flavourings to processed cheese.

Generally speaking, cheese consists of approximately one-third protein, one-third fat and one-third water. In addition, it contains calcium and vitamin A from the milk and the salt which is added during manufacture. It is thus an excellent body-building, energy and protective food and has the additional merit of being relatively cheap. The fact that its fat and protein are so intimately mixed together makes it rather difficult to digest. For this reason cheese should be chewed well and in the case of young children, finely shredded or grated. If cheese is cooked it should not be overheated, otherwise the protein will be over-coagulated and made more difficult to digest. Cheese should be eaten along with carbohydrate foods, e.g., bread and biscuits. In this way the fat of the cheese is more completely oxidised in the body and its protein increases the value of the protein in the bread and biscuits.

Skimmed and Separated Milks

Skimmed and separated milks are the liquids left after the cream has been skimmed off or separated. They still contain the other ingredients of milk and are valuable foods, particularly for their animal protein, riboflavin and calcium and should not be wasted. Such milks are very useful in making bread, cakes and scones. Large quantities are sold in a dried form. Skimmed and separated milks are not suitable foods for infants as they lack fat.

Buttermilk

Buttermilk is the waste product of butter manufacture. It contains the constituents of the original milk, except the fat, and is distinctly acid due to the action of lactic acid bacteria. It is useful in making scones. The food value of the scones is increased, and the lactic acid releases carbon dioxide from the bicarbonate of soda used in the scones and thus aerates them. Dried buttermilk powders are sold for use in breadmaking.

Whey

Whey is the liquid left after the removal of the curd when milk has been curdled by rennet or by souring with an acid such as vinegar, or by bacteria. The casein and fat are removed in the curd and the whey contains only small amounts of food material, chiefly the proteins, lactalbumen and lactoglobulin, and milk sugar. It is usually used for feeding farm animals although a dried whey powder can be bought for confectionery purposes.

Evaporated Milk

Is milk from which one-third of the water has been removed. The milk is first pasteurised, then the water is removed by evaporation at a low pressure (to avoid having to heat the milk to a high temperature). The concentrated milk is then homogenised, canned and sterilised. Sometimes this milk is irradiated, which will convert some of the ergosterol to vitamin D. The heat treatment destroys vitamin C and some vitamin B_1, it also alters some of the proteins and the taste is changed. The homogenisation and the change in the proteins makes evaporated milk more digestible than normal cows' milk.

Condensed Milk

Condensed milk is made by evaporating away about two-thirds of the water from either full cream or separated milk. The condensed milk is then sweetened. The addition of sugar improves the flavour, increases the energy value and checks bacterial action. Whether full cream or separated, the condensed milk is hermetically sealed in sterilised tins. The tins must have a label attached giving a clear description of the contents.

Condensed milks, as a result of their heat treatment and storage in sealed tins, contain fewer bacteria than fresh milk and are less likely to spread infectious diseases. Provided they are kept sealed they will keep indefinitely. Condensed sweetened skimmed milks are deficient in fat and quite unsuitable for infants. Sweetened condensed full cream milk contains too much sugar which is liable to upset an infant's digestion. Mixing this type of condensed milk with water to give a more correct proportion of sugar makes the proteins and fat deficient.

Composition of Typical Condensed Milks

Percentage	*Whole, Sweetened*	*Whole, Unsweetened*	*Skimmed, Sweetened*
Protein	8·2	8·5	9·5
Fat	9·2	9·2	0·5
Carbohydrate	49·6	11·5	55·8
Calcium	0·3	0·3	0·3

Milk Powders

These are prepared by the removal of practically the whole of the water of milk. They are produced from both whole milk and separated milk. The milk is first homogenised. It is then dried by either the roller process or the spray process, see p. 160.

Provided they are kept dry in airtight containers, milk powders will keep indefinitely. The fat of dried whole milk is liable to go rancid on exposure to air. Dried whole milk powder contains all the ingredients of milk in a concentrated form. Dried skimmed milk contains no fat and consequently no vitamin A or vitamin D but contains the whole of the protein, calcium and riboflavin of the milk. It is valuable in cooking and baking but should not be used to totally replace full cream milk.

Composition of Typical Milk Powders

Percentage	*Whole milk powder*	*Skimmed milk powder*
Protein	25·6	35·8
Fat	26·7	0·7
Carbohydrate	35·6	47·9
Calcium	0·9	1·2

Patent Baby-Foods

Dried whole milk is made the basis of patent baby-foods. It is frequently modified in some way, e.g., by adding sugar, removing fat, adding vitamins and iron, to make it more closely resemble human milk in composition. It is then said to be "humanised."

Fermented Milks (Yoghurt)

The process of fermentation is one of the oldest methods known of preserving or improving the nutritive constituents of milk. In spite of the fact that modern methods have made fermentation of milk unnecessary, there is a growing demand for fermented milks, principally because of the claims put forward as to their exceptional health-giving properties. The principal types of fermented milks are kephyr, koumiss and yoghurt, the last being the commonest in this country.

Yoghurt is a thick, curdled milk which is decidedly acid. It is a nourishing and refreshing food which is easily digested. Milk is converted into yoghurt by curdling it with special bacterial cultures. The acidity of yoghurt is due to the formation of lactic acid from lactose, and the digestibility to the partial peptonisation of the casein.

The milk used for the manufacture of yoghurt is usually skimmed milk; fruit, flavourings and sometimes vitamins may be added to it.

11 Meat, Fish and Eggs

MEAT

The term "meat" includes the flesh and some of the internal organs (offal) of animals and birds. The chief animals used in this country as sources of meat are the bullock (beef), sheep (lamb and mutton), pig (pork) and rabbit. The chief birds are domestic poultry, such as chickens, ducks, geese and turkeys, and game birds such as the pheasant, partridge and grouse.

Flesh, or lean meat, consists of muscle tissue which is built up of microscopic fibres. These fibres are arranged in bundles which are held together by connective tissue of a gristle-like nature. These bundles are again grouped into bigger bundles surrounded by connective tissue and the whole muscle surrounded by a sheath of connective tissue which merges at each end into gristle or tendons joining the muscle to bone. Dispersed throughout the fibres are nerves and bloodvessels and embedded in the connective tissue between the fibres is a certain amount of fat.

Muscle fibres vary considerably in length and thickness and in the amounts of connective tissue, gristle and fat they contain. It is upon these variations that the tenderness of meat very largely depends. In the flesh of older animals the muscle fibres are thick and long and have a large amount of connective tissue and gristle. It is thus tougher than the flesh of younger animals with thinner, shorter fibres, less connective tissue and less gristle. Even in the same animal the muscles which have had most work to do are stronger and tougher and have more connective tissue and gristle than muscles from other parts of its body which have had less work to do. This explains, for instance, why shin beef, which is the leg muscle of the bullock, is tougher than sirloin which comes from the muscles of its back. In the same way, chicken leg is tougher than the breast.

The amount of fat in the connective tissue varies with the kind of animal and between animals of the same kind according to their

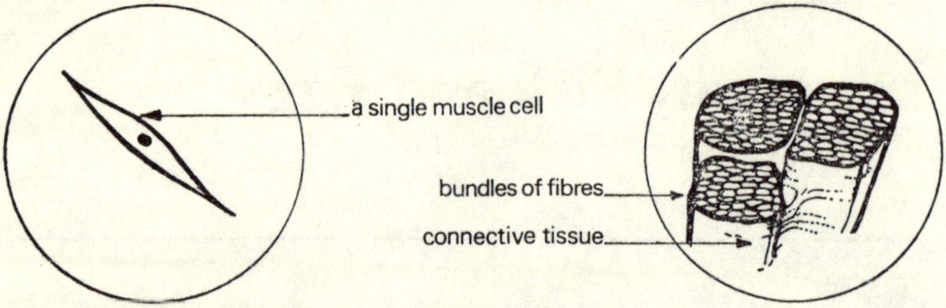

Meat: single muscle cell and bundles of fibres.

age and food. Most forms of game contain very little fat. Beef contains more than veal while pork contains more than beef or mutton. Water birds such as ducks and geese contain more fat in their muscle fibres than land birds such as chickens and turkeys. A large amount of fat tends to make the meat less easily digested by preventing the digestive juices coming into contact with the fibres. It should be made clear that the fat referred to here is not the fat deposited under the animal's skin and round its internal organs such as the kidneys. It is sometimes called "invisible" fat because it cannot be seen with the naked eye.

Each microscopic muscle fibre contains water in which are dissolved proteins, mineral salts and substances known as "extractives." The chief protein is *myosinogen* which clots into *myosin* when the animal is killed and its body cools. This causes the muscle fibres to go hard and accounts for the stiffening after death known as *rigor mortis*. In this condition the meat is very tough and must be hung until the rigor mortis has passed off. Gradually, the coagulated myosin liquefies because of the formation of acids and the action of enzymes in the fibres. The meat thus becomes tender and the acids improve the flavour and help to break down the connective tissue. In the case of game, the hanging is carried out until it is "high," that is, until it has begun to putrefy. These effects are sometimes imitated artificially by soaking tough meat in vinegar and water for a short time.

The mineral salts in the muscle fibres are chiefly phosphates. There is iron in the haemoglobin of any blood left in the meat but not much of it is "available" in digestion. Muscle fibres contain very little calcium.

The extractives are so called because they can be extracted from meat by boiling it in water. It is these substances which give meat its flavour and the variation in taste between different kinds of meat is due largely to differences in the kind and amount of extractives they contain. The extractives powerfully stimulate the flow of digestive juices and thus help in the digestion of meat. They have no actual food value.

Connective tissue has two kinds of fibres; one kind is composed of a protein known as *collagen*, the other kind of a quite different protein *elastin*. Both are quite different from the protein myosin. Elastin is insoluble in water and very tough. Collagen is also insoluble in water but moist heat converts it into *gelatine*. This conversion takes place during the cooking of meat. The meat is thus made more tender and the digestive juices are better able to come into contact with the myosin of the muscle fibres. The pounding of beef steak with a stick before cooking breaks open the sheaths of connective tissue and produces a similar effect. For the same reason, meat should be carved across the length of the fibres and not along them.

The vitamins in lean meat are chiefly those of the B group, particularly riboflavin and nicotinic acid. Lean meat is not a rich source of thiamine, although lean pork, bacon and ham are exceptions. This is probably due to the fact that the food of foreign pigs (maize) contains more thiamine than that of cattle and sheep. Lean meat contains traces of vitamin A in its "invisible" fat, but very little ascorbic acid is found in meat.

OFFAL

The internal organs are usually referred to as "offal." The main offal foods are liver, kidneys and tripe.

Liver and kidneys are more compact and have less connective tissue than lean meat. They consist chiefly of proteins with a little fat. Their proteins are different from those of lean meat. They are called nucleo-proteins and are liable to form uric acid on digestion. For this reason, these foods should be avoided by persons suffering from gout. Both of them, and particularly liver, contain large amounts of vitamin A and iron. Consequently both are valuable protective foods.

Tripe is prepared from the stomach and intestines of cattle and sheep. It contains a large amount of connective tissue which is changed into gelatine during the long slow cooking it undergoes.

The fact that it contains no extractives makes it lacking in flavour but it can be made palatable by serving with sauce or, better still, with milk and onions. Tripe is a valuable and easily digested food. In addition to protein, it contains an appreciable quantity of calcium from the lime used in its preparation.

POULTRY

The application of industrial-type farming to the rearing of poultry has led to a dramatic drop in the cost of chickens, but other types of poultry are still generally rather expensive.

Chicken has less fat and iron than beef, but it is richer in protein, calcium and nicotinic acid. Because of its fine texture and the absence of fat, chicken is a very easily digested food rich in high quality protein. Turkey has a similar food value.

Duck and goose are both still luxury foods and traditionally are thought of as being very fatty. In fact the fat content of roast duck and goose is similar to that of roast beef.

MEAT EXTRACTS

Meat extracts are made by treating fresh meat with boiling water to dissolve out its soluble ingredients. These include minerals, extractives and the vitamins nicotinic acid and riboflavin. The extract is concentrated to give the thick brown material with a strong "meaty" smell which we all know.

Because of the minerals and extractives they contain, soups and beverages made from meat extracts give flavour and help digestion by stimulating the flow of digestive juices. They contain no protein and no fat and so are neither body-builders nor energy foods and it is an exaggeration to say that they contain all the goodness of meat in a concentrated form. They do, however, contain a large amount of nicotinic acid and a fairly large amount of riboflavin. It is in these two vitamins that their main food value lies, but only small quantities are normally used.

SOUPS AND BEEF TEA

It will now be realised that the water in which meat has been cooked will contain minerals, extractives, nicotinic acid and riboflavin. Soups and beef tea will thus contain all these materials and if the meat itself is added the soup or beef tea will provide protein. Any vegetables or cereals added will also increase the food value but long heating will destroy any ascorbic acid the vegetables might contain. The real value of soups is as stimulants to the appetite and as aids to digestion by increasing the flow of digestive juices. This is why it is customary to take soup at the beginning of dinner.

CHARACTERISTICS OF FRESH MEAT

If meat is fresh it will have the following characteristics:

(1) It will be firm and elastic to the touch.
(2) The colour will be bright.
(3) It will be moist but not wet.
(4) The flesh will be mottled with fat.
(5) The fat will be pale yellow in colour and of firm texture.

For the cooking of meat see Chapter 16. For the preservation of meat see Chapter 15.

FISH

As with meat, the chief food materials in fish are protein and fat. Compared with meat, fish contains very much more waste material in the form of skin, head and bones and a larger amount of water. The connective tissue of fish contains collagen only without any of the tough elastin. This collagen is easily converted into gelatine during the cooking of fish. This explains why fish is more tender than meat and more easily cooked. The fat in fish is found entirely dispersed among the muscle fibres: there is no separate fatty tissue as there is in meat. The amounts of minerals and extractives are much less than in meat and this accounts for their comparative lack of flavour. As a result, fish eaten too frequently is apt to become insipid and monotonous unless attractively cooked and served. Well-made sauces, vinegar, pepper and salt are valuable aids in making fish more appetising.

The flesh, i.e., the muscle of fish, is divided into flakes between the bones. In some fish, e.g., cod, the flakes are large and easily separated from the bones, while in others, e.g., herrings, they are small and difficult to remove. The proteins of the muscle fibres are similar to those of meat. They contain the essential amino-acids and are of high biological value.

The amount of fat in fish varies very considerably with the type of fish and the time of the year. Herrings, mackerel, pilchards, and sardines contain up to 20%, and are known as *fat fish.* The actual amount of fat in fish alters with the time of year because it depends upon the fish's food and the nearness of spawning. Herrings contain most fat during the summer months when they are feeding intensively and least in spring and autumn when they are spawning. The salmon is at its best when it first leaves the sea to go upstream to breed. During the breeding season the fat is used up and the flesh becomes pale and watery.

Fish which never contain much fat are known as *white fish.* They include cod, halibut, haddock, plaice, sole, hake, turbot and whiting.

The mineral salts in fish consist chiefly of calcium and phosphorus. These are provided in largest amounts when we eat the bones of such fish as sardines, sprats and whitebait. Sea fish contain valuable traces of iodine but there is very little iron in fish except in sardines and sprats. Fat fish contain the fat-soluble vitamins A and D. In fact, herrings, sardines, mackerel and salmon are among the few good food sources of vitamin D. White fish contain only a small amount of vitamin A and no vitamin D at all except that stored up in the liver. Fish liver oils, particularly those of halibut and cod, contain exceptionally large amounts of both vitamins.

There are small amounts of the B vitamins in most fish; fat fish containing more than white. Fat fish are thus very valuable body-building, energy and protective foods while white fish are body-building foods only.

Because of the short fibres and small amount of connective tissue the flesh of white fish is amongst our most valuable and easily digested animal foods. Fat fish, as we have seen, are even more nutritious but their fat makes them less easy to digest, particularly for invalids. For normal healthy persons leading an active life herrings, and other fat fish, are amongst our finest and cheapest foods for protein, fat and vitamins A and D. Their frequent use in the diet cannot be too highly recommended.

FISH OFFALS

The only offal of fish which is ordinarily eaten is the *roe.* "Hard roe," in which the eggs are easily visible, is the ovary of the female fish. "Soft roe," or milt, is the corresponding organ in the male fish. Both consist largely of protein with small amounts of fat. *Caviare* is the salted roe of the sturgeon.

Fish goes bad very quickly and for this reason should be very fresh and cooked as soon as possible. Whether fish is purchased whole, or in fillets or steaks, the flesh should be firm and without disagreeable smell. In the case of whole fish, the gills should be examined to see if they are bright and clear and the eyes should be bright and full and not dull and sunken.

For the cooking of fish see Chapter 16. For the preservation of fish see Chapter 15.

SHELL FISH

Included under this heading are the *crustaceans*, crab and lobster, and the *molluscs*, oysters, mussels, winkles and cockles.

The flesh of lobster and crab is found in the claws and tail. The body consists mainly of liver. The flesh is dense and coarse with thick fibre walls which make it rather indigestible. Their food value consists in their protein and fat. Prawns and shrimps are similar.

The use of vinegar with these shell fish helps to soften the muscle fibres besides adding to the flavour.

Oysters, mussels, winkles and cockles contain small amounts of protein, fat and minerals, including iodine and iron.

In both crustaceans and molluscs there is always a very large amount of waste on account of the shell. They are best regarded as occasional tasty delicacies.

Those shellfish which are eaten raw must be correctly washed and absolutely fresh. All shellfish goes bad very quickly and care in purchasing, cooking and storage is essential.

EGGS

By the term eggs we ordinarily mean those of the domestic fowl but these are not the only edible eggs. The eggs of such domestic birds as ducks, geese and turkeys as well as those of such wild birds as the plover, gull and heron can also be used as human food. Other eggs used for food are those of the turtle and many varieties of fish, e.g., herring (roe) and sturgeon (caviare). For our purpose we shall confine ourselves to the hen's egg which constitutes the chief source of our supply of eggs.

We shall better understand the value of an egg as food if we realise that it is a living organism. It contains an undeveloped chick, or embryo, with its store of food enclosed in a protective shell. The fact that the living chicken steps out of the egg shell when the egg hatches after twenty-one days sitting or incubation shows us that the egg must contain every type of food material necessary for its rapid growth and development. We should expect to find that it contains proteins and minerals for building the flesh and bones of the rapidly growing embryo and fat to supply energy. Fat is a more compact fuel than carbohydrate and thus more suitable for storing in a confined space such as an egg. The vitamins we should expect to find will be vitamins A and D since these are the ones most closely concerned with growth. All these expectations are borne out in fact.

The shell consists chiefly of chalk (calcium carbonate) with small amounts of calcium phosphate. It is not a solid shell forming a hermetic seal but is pitted with tiny holes. In other words, it is porous. This allows air to pass into the interior of the egg for the living embryo to breathe in oxygen. The carbon dioxide it breathes out passes outwards through the pores of the shell. Unfortunately, the porous character of the shell allows bacteria to enter the egg and moisture to escape. When eggs are stored the contents are liable to go bad through the action of these bacteria and to shrink owing to the loss of moisture.

Underneath the shell is a thin parchment-like *shell-membrane* which divides at the broad end of the egg into two layers to form an *air chamber*. Inside the shell membrane are the *white* and the *yolk*. The white is a sticky liquid in layers of varying thickness. The yolk is roughly spherical in shape and is surrounded by a thin elastic membrane. Underneath this *yolk membrane* is the *living embryo* which can be seen as a small circular disc. Attached to the yolk are two fibrous twisted cords, known as *chalazas* or balancers which hold the yolk in position and prevent injury to the embryo by acting as "shock-absorbers" when the egg is moved.

The white consists essentially of a solution in water of proteins, mainly *egg albumen* or *ovalbumen*. It also contains some riboflavin. Unlike the protein of meat and fish, that of eggs is not in the form of muscle fibres and is not surrounded by tough connective

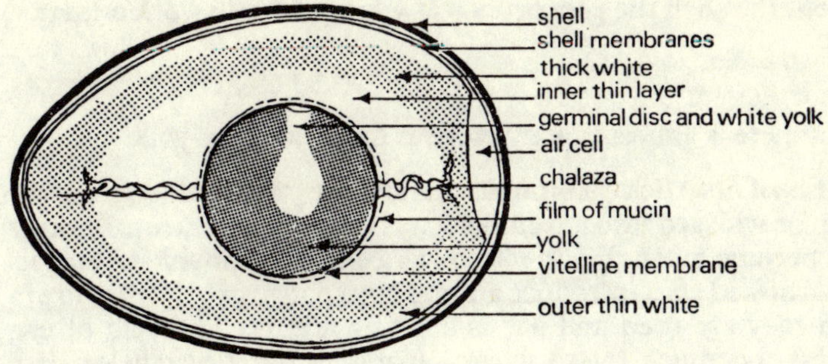

Diagram of fowl's egg.

tissue. It is in a colloidal solution and is thus easily digested, and very suitable for young children, invalids and convalescents.

The yolk is the chief storehouse of food for the young chick. It is very much richer and more complex than the white. It contains less water, more protein and a large proportion of fat and minerals. In addition to ovalbumen, the yolk contains two other proteins, *vitellin*, which contains phosphorus, and *livetin*. The fats in egg yolk are highly emulsified and, consequently, easily digested. A fat-like substance *lecithin*, which contains phosphorus, is also present. The minerals include valuable calcium, iron and sulphur in addition to the phosphorus already mentioned. The vitamins include vitamins A and D in the fats with some thiamine and riboflavin. The yolk is thus an exceptionally fine food with its animal protein, its easily digested fat, its valuable calcium, iron, sulphur and phosphorus, and its vitamins.

Eggs are highly nutritious foods which are also easily digested and absorbed and are widely used in baking and cooking. When used as a main dish, two eggs should replace a portion of meat or fish.

The average weight of a hen's egg is about sixty grammes and its approximate composition is as follows:

Shell and membrane	10·1%
White	59·7%
Yolk	30·2%

Without the shell the proportions of white and yolk work out at:

White	66·4%
Yolk	33·6%

so that there is almost exactly twice as much white as yolk.

Because of its sticky glutinous nature the white of egg can be beaten or whisked into a froth which is almost permanent. Bubbles of air become entangled in its substance and are unable to escape. Thus whisked eggs introduce air into any sponge or cake mixture in which they are used and act as aerating agents. The yolk of egg contains too much fat to whisk separately but nevertheless is a valuable ingredient in baked foods. It improves their colour, flavour and food value and its fat has a "shortening" and moistening action. The best results are obtained by using the whole egg for baking purposes. As a general rule, a whole egg can aerate an equal weight of flour, i.e., 4 eggs to 120 grammes flour. If less than this proportion is used baking powder or self-raising flour will be needed.

In addition to their use directly as foods, and as aerating and enriching agents in sponge and cake mixtures, eggs are used in omelettes, custards, and Yorkshire and other puddings. Egg whites are used separately in meringues, macaroons, dessert biscuits and royal icing.

When eggs are heated their proteins set or coagulate. This coagulation begins at about 60° C so that fully boiling water (100° C,) is not essential to the "boiling" of an egg. The same coagulation takes place in other methods of cooking eggs, e.g., frying, scrambling and poaching. As a result of the coagulation of the proteins the whole egg solidifies. The white becomes a soft, tough mass but the yolk, because of its fat, breaks up into a powder. The higher the temperature and the longer the time of cooking the tougher and more solid the eggs become and, therefore, more difficult to digest. Thus, fried eggs are harder to digest than poached or scrambled eggs, and hard-boiled eggs more difficult to digest than lightly boiled ones.

This same coagulation of the proteins takes place when mixtures containing eggs are cooked or baked. In sponge and cake mixtures it helps to fix the sponge or cake in shape during baking. In sauces, egg custards and lemon cheese it helps the stiffening which takes place on cooling. In the case of these articles care must be taken to mix the ingredients thoroughly and not to heat them too strongly or the proteins will harden into lumps and "curdle" the mixture. The mixture should, therefore, not be permitted to boil after the egg is added. The use of a double pan is advisable.

The use of eggs for binding mixtures together is explained in the same way. When the proteins coagulate on heating they bind together the loose or dry ingredients, e.g., in rissoles and croquettes. The use of eggs on the outside of fried foods which might fall apart in cooking is also due to the same action. The proteins set on the outside during the cooking and prevent the foods from breaking, and also prevent too much fat being soaked up by the mixture. Bread crumbs are used after the egg has been applied to give a crisp brown appearance.

When eggs are to be kept for some time they should be placed in a suitable tray with the blunt ends, containing the air-chamber, uppermost. In this way the yolk is kept in its proper position completely surrounded by the white. The white is less likely to deteriorate into the condition known as "watery" white. Of the two parts of an egg the white is less easily attacked by bacteria than the yolk with its richer food store and, when it completely surrounds the yolk, the white helps to protect it. The eggs should be placed in a cool dry place away from any strong-smelling foods. Eggs readily absorb odours and their taste is thus spoiled.

If eggs are good for us, they are unfortunately also good for bacteria, which multiply in them rapidly and spoil the contents. The sulphur compounds of the proteins give sulphuretted hydrogen on decomposition and it is this gas which gives the unpleasant smell to a rotten egg. Another cause which renders eggs unsuitable for human food is the partial growth of the embryo due to irregular collection or accidental incubation. Since the contents of the egg are enclosed in a mineral shell it is impossible to know by looking at it whether the egg is fresh or bad until the shell is broken, when it is sometimes only too obvious that things are not as they should be. Some simple method of testing the quality and freshness of a whole egg is obviously desirable, and two methods are in common use. These tests are the brine test and the candling test.

The brine test consists in placing the egg in a 10% salt solution in a tall jar, and is a simple and infallible test. A newly laid egg will sink in such a solution and lie flat at the bottom of the jar. An older egg will have lost weight by evaporation of water through its porous shell, and the consequent drying and shrinking of the contents will have enlarged the air chamber. As a result, the egg will become lighter and more buoyant with age. A two-day-old egg will float near the bottom of the solution with its broad end upwards. A three-day-old egg will float about half-way up the solution, and one five days old or more will float on the surface. Thus the older the egg the nearer the surface it will float. While it is not always possible to judge the age of an egg by this method, it is easy to decide whether an egg is fresh or not.

The candling test is dependent upon the transparency of eggs to light. It is a quicker method and more suitable for use in egg-packing stations than the brine test but requires skill and experience to obtain reliable results. The apparatus consists of a lamp surrounded by a metal shade bored with a hole. The egg to be tested is placed against the hole, slowly turned between finger and thumb, and the transparency of the egg observed. As the contents of the egg dry and shrink with age they become more and more opaque.

EGG SUBSTITUTES

We have already seen that the use of eggs in baking is chiefly as aerators and that the white of egg is the part which whips up into a froth and entangles air bubbles in its sticky glutinous substance. These air bubbles are retained in the cake or sponge mixture until they are baked and so make it light, i.e., aerate them. Many cheap *egg substitutes* are manufactured which simulate the aerating power of egg white. These substitutes generally contain starch, bicarbonate of soda, tartaric acid and some glutinous substance such as gelatine. The mixture is given an egg-like appearance by the addition to it of some yellow colouring. The mixture is similar to baking powder and when mixed with water, carbon dioxide is given off which is retained by the glutinous substance and the mixture beats up in a similar way to genuine egg. Such substitutes are, however, very much inferior to eggs as aerating and strengthening agents and are in no way comparable with eggs in food value. Their only merit is their cheapness.

Custard powders may be similar in composition to egg substitutes as given above, or may merely consist of cornflour, or other forms of starch, coloured to resemble egg and flavoured, usually with vanilla. When mixed with a little cold milk to a paste, then stirred with boiling milk, the custard powder sets on cooling owing to the formation of a thick starch paste. They do not compare in food value with genuine egg custard made from eggs and milk but have the merit of the milk used in their preparation.

The preservation of eggs is discussed in Chapter 15.

In concluding this important chapter there is one other point about meat, fish and eggs which we wish to point out. These three foods contain little or no carbohydrates. It is for this reason that they are normally eaten with some food rich in starch, e.g., potatoes, bread and flour. In this way they are made more complete foods.

12 Beverages

We have already seen in Chapter 5 that nearly three-quarters of the body consists of water and that water is essential for the digestion and absorption of our food and for its transport throughout the body. We have seen, too, that water is continually being lost from the body through the skin in perspiration, the lungs as water vapour in expired air, the kidneys in urine and the bowels in faeces. This daily loss amounts to an average of about four and a quarter pints which must be made good. We may replace this lost water as drink, in foods, or by the water formed by the oxidation of foods in the body. It was stated on page 44 that the average amount of water required as drink is about 1½ litres. This includes, in addition to water itself, such fluids as tea, coffee, cocoa, mineral waters, alcoholic beverages and so on.

WATER

Water itself is the best and most natural drink and the finest thirst quencher. What little taste water possesses is due to the presence in it of dissolved oxygen and carbon dioxide and dissolved mineral salts such as calcium bicarbonate and calcium and magnesium sulphates. The effect of dissolved oxygen and carbon dioxide is easily realised when well-aerated water is contrasted with boiled water from which the dissolved gases have been expelled by heat. Of the dissolved mineral salts, the calcium bicarbonate of temporarily hard water gives a pleasanter taste than the calcium and magnesium sulphates of permanently hard water. Very soft water has less taste than harder water with its dissolved mineral salts and is more likely to dissolve small amounts of lead from lead piping and may thus be harmful to health. It may even taste acid or peaty if coming off moorland gathering grounds. Hard water supplies quite a useful amount of calcium to the diet.

NATURAL MINERAL WATERS

The waters from natural springs in many parts of the world, e.g.,

Apollinaris, Perrier, Seltzer and Vichy, contain comparatively large amounts of dissolved carbon dioxide and various mineral salts such as salt, bicarbonates of soda, lime and magnesia. In the past, exaggerated claims have been made for their medicinal value in the cure of gout, rheumatoid arthritis and other diseases. The Victorian cult of visiting various "spas" to "drink the waters" appears almost to have died out. Most of these waters are sparkling because of their carbon dioxide and slightly alkaline because of their dissolved carbonates. It is probably true to say that the carbon dioxide will stimulate the flow of gastric juice and the alkalinity will partly neutralise the acidity of gastric juice but not much more than that can be said of them.

ARTIFICIAL MINERAL WATERS

Artificial imitations of natural mineral waters can be purchased which consist of solutions of various carbonates in spring water or distilled water. For example, soda water contains a little bicarbonate of soda, magnesia water, magnesium carbonate and seltzer water, common salt, bicarbonate of soda, magnesium carbonate and hydrochloric acid and is heavily charged with carbon dioxide. Much so-called "soda" water is merely water containing carbon dioxide dissolved under pressure. It is really "carbonated" water and contains no soda whatever.

Sweetened and flavoured mineral waters comprise lemonade, orangeade, "ginger beer," and so on. These consist of water sweetened with sugar, made tart by the addition of an acid such as acetic, citric or phosphoric, flavoured to resemble the material after which they are named and finally charged with carbon dioxide under pressure to make them effervesce. It is unusual for them to contain the natural fruit acids, citric and tartaric, or the natural fruit flavourings. Genuine fermented ginger beer is an exception and does contain natural ginger and, as a result of fermentation, some alcohol too.

FRUIT JUICES

Juices expressed from fruits by specially designed machines and canned, or bottled and pasteurised are pleasant to drink and contain the sugar and acids of the original fruits as well as a small proportion of ascorbic acid. These are very different from the artificial lemonade, orangeade and so on and are definitely beneficial. Large amounts are drunk in the U.S.A. and their use in this country is increasing.

The latest development is the concentration of fruit juices by evaporation under low pressure followed by preservation by deep-freezing. When suitably diluted with water these frozen concentrated fruit juices have the same vitamin C content as the fresh juice. Sometimes sugar is added to the juices which of course raises their kcal value.

TEA

Tea has been used as a beverage in China at least since 2700 B.C. It was introduced into this country early in the Stuart period but it was not until 1660 that it came to the notice of Pepys.

Tea consists of the dried leaves of a shrub, *Camellia thea*, grown in China, India, Sri Lanka, Java and Japan. Originally all the tea in this country came from China but we now import most of our tea from India and Sri Lanka and very little from China.

The tea plant is a hardy evergreen which is kept down by severe pruning to a low shrub of convenient height for hand plucking. The leaves are plucked at intervals during the season. The size of the leaf varies according to age and position on the twig and determines the grade of tea. The smaller, younger leaves and buds at the tops of the twigs are the finest grade and the larger, older, tougher leaves lower down the lowest grade.

The process of manufacture is briefly as follows:

(1) *Withering*
The leaves are spread on hessian mats for several hours until about half the water is dried out.

(2) *Rolling*
The leaves are rolled by machine or hand to break open the cells to release the juice and bring about the twist in the leaves.

(3) *Fermentation*
The rolled leaves are spread for several hours on cement tables with free access of cool air to ferment or oxidise. Oxidation of some of the tannin and development of the essential oils are responsible for the flavour. The colour of the leaves changes to a bright coppery shade during fermentation. Light fermentation gives flavour and pungency; longer fermentation gives strength and

body. If fermented too long, tea becomes sour. Green tea is not fermented.

(4) *Firing*

Fermentation is stopped by drying the leaves in currents of hot air.

Tea is generally imported into this country as "originals" or unblended tea and afterwards blended by professional tea tasters to suit the needs of various districts dependent mainly upon the hardness or softness of the local drinking water. Hard water tends to make a thin tea and soft water to make it more coloured.

Tea contains a useful amount of fluorine and small amounts of other mineral salts and riboflavin. Otherwise it has little food value other than that of the cream or milk and sugar taken with it. The caffeine it contains is a mild nervous stimulant with no harmful after effects. It is speedily dissolved in boiling water. The tannin of tea is an astringent which exercises an inhibitory action on the intestinal tract, and coagulates protein and so checks digestion. Tannin is not readily soluble in boiling water but is extracted on standing and gives a bitter flavour to tea. The essential oils of tea give it its aroma and pungency. China tea has the most delicate flavour, most caffeine and least tannin. Indian and Sri Lanka teas have more body, colour and tannin.

In the correct brewing of tea the maximum amount of caffeine and essential oil should be extracted and the minimum amount of tannin. This is best achieved by the following method:

(1) Pour hot water into a teapot and leave to stand until thoroughly hot.

(2) Pour off this water and put in the tea, allowing two level teaspoons for each 250 ml of water.

(3) Bring the water to the boil and pour *immediately* over the tea. Water which has been long boiled loses its dissolved gases and gives a flat, insipid tea.

(4) Allow the tea to stand (infuse) for three to four minutes only. Stir well before pouring out. This length of time is sufficient to extract the caffeine and essential oils. Long infusion extracts the tannin and gives a bitter taste.

(5) Serve at once.

(6) If a second cup per person is required, pour fresh boiling water on the tea leaves and infuse again. This second brewing will be weaker and inferior in flavour.

(7) The milk or cream should be poured into the cups before the tea. The milk helps to precipitate any tannin present.

COFFEE

Coffee was introduced into this country in 1652 and quickly became the vogue in "coffee houses." In most parts of the world, except the United Kingdom, coffee is the most popular beverage.

The coffee plant is an evergreen shrub grown in the moist tropics, chiefly Arabia, East Africa, Ethiopia, India, Sri Lanka, Java, Jamaica and Brazil. The fruit or coffee cherry consists of an outer skin, a pulp, and a "stone" with a parchment skin enclosing two seeds ("beans" or "berries"). The stone is dried, the husk removed and the berries roasted before use. The roasting makes the berries brittle and easily ground, caramelises some of the sugar and develops aroma and flavour. As soon as roasted, the berries should be quickly cooled and afterwards kept in an airtight container. Roasting should be done frequently, even daily, and preferably followed by immediate grinding. The aroma and flavour quickly disappear after grinding, particularly if the ground coffee is not kept enclosed, because of the very volatile character of the essential oils.

To make coffee in the home the simplest way is to use an earthenware jug with a lip for pouring and a lid. The method is as follows:

(1) Warm the jug with boiling water. When thoroughly hot, pour out the water and put in at least 25 g of coffee for every $\frac{1}{2}$ litre of liquor required.

(2) Pour in freshly boiling water and stir well with a wooden spoon.

(3) Allow to infuse in a warm place for about ten minutes.

(4) Strain and serve very hot.

(5) Milk, when used with coffee, should be hot but not boiling.

Alternative methods of making coffee involve the use of special drip coffee pots, vacuum coffee pots or coffee percolators. It is doubtful if the resulting coffee is in any way better than, or even as good as, that produced in a jug by the method outlined above.

Coffee contains a much smaller amount of caffeine than tea but more tannin. It acts upon the nervous system which it stimulates, so causing wakefulness. It may also have an aperient action by stimulating the muscles of the intestines, hence its place at the end of dinner.

Coffee is frequently mixed with chicory which is the dried powdery root of the wild endive. Roasted chicory contains no caffeine but contains easily soluble colouring matters, including caramel.

Coffee essence. This is made by evaporating coffee, usually mixed with chicory, and often with added synthetic flavouring.

Coffee powders. These are made by brewing coffee and then drying the filtered liquid. The liquid may either be spray-dried, which produces a powder with much of the original flavour but no odour; or freeze-dried, which produces granules with much of the original flavour and aroma.

COCOA

Cocoa first came to this country about 1650. It is obtained from a small evergreen tree, *Cacao theobroma*. The fruits resemble the marrow or cucumber and have a similar soft pulpy case in which the seeds are embedded. The seeds are removed from the fruit and roasted and the roasted seeds separated into two parts known as cocoa nibs. The nibs are ground between hot rollers to form a semi-liquid mass from which the greater part of the fat is extracted as cocoa butter. The remaining cocoa is run into moulds to cool and set as cocoa cake which is further ground and sifted to form cocoa powder.

The stimulant in cocoa is theobromine which is similar to the caffeine of tea and coffee but much milder in its action on the nervous system. In addition, cocoa contains some tannin, fat, starch, protein, B vitamins and mineral salts (in particular iron) so that cocoa has considerable food value. The small amounts of cocoa used daily, however, do not make any significant addition to the diet. It is as a substance which makes palatable the drinking of hot water or milk that cocoa is justified as a beverage. Because of its mild stimulant and the food value of the added milk and sugar, it is the most suitable of the common beverages for children.

Cocoa is best made as follows:

(1) Allow two level teaspoons of cocoa for 250 ml of milk or milk and water. Add sugar to taste.

(2) Mix cocoa, sugar and some of the cold liquid to a smooth paste.

(3) Boil the remaining liquid and pour into the cocoa and sugar.

(4) Return the mixture to the pan and boil for one or two minutes before serving. This second boiling cooks the starch in the cocoa and greatly improves the flavour.

Although they are food-drinks rather than beverages, it is convenient to mention here such proprietary articles as Ovaltine and Bournvita which consist of malt extract, milk, eggs, and cocoa. With the milk taken with them they are nutritious, easily digested and very suitable for invalids, convalescents and children.

ALCOHOLIC BEVERAGES

Alcoholic beverages are made by the fermentation of glucose into alcohol and carbon dioxide together with small amounts of other by-products such as acids and esters which affect the flavour and body of the beverage. Different beverages are produced according to the foodstuff fermented by the yeast, e.g., wine from grapes, cider from apples and beer from malt. The amount of alcohol in such beverages depends mainly upon the amount of fermentable sugar present in the original foodstuff. The amounts of alcohol in spirits such as whisky, brandy, rum and gin are increased by distillation and in liqueurs the spirits are sweetened with sugar and flavoured with various herbs and fruit peels. Fortified wines such as port have spirit added to them.

BEERS

The starting point in the production of beer is the preparation of a "mash" of malt in water. Malt is made by soaking barley grains in water and then spreading them on the floor of a malt house and keeping them at a moderate temperature. Under these conditions the barley grains germinate and the diastase formed by the embryos transforms some of the starch of the endosperms into dextrins and maltose (malt sugar). The sprouted grains are then dried in a malt kiln. The dried malt is ground and a mash made of it with water. The dextrins and maltose and small amounts of other soluble substances from the malt pass into solution. The liquid or wort is strained from the malt, boiled with hops which have a flavouring and antiseptic action, cooled and then fermented by specially cultivated yeast in large vats. After fermentation the yeast is skimmed off and the beer pumped into barrels. Slow fermentation continues in the barrels and the beer becomes aerated since the carbon dioxide formed is unable to escape.

Porter and stout are also made from malt and hops but the malt is first roasted in cylinders. This results in the conversion of some of the maltose into caramel and gives these beverages their darker colour and special flavour.

Beer, porter and stout contain from 3–6% alcohol, some dextrins and sugars, riboflavin and nicotinic acid. Consequently, these beverages have a certain amount of food value.

WINES

In the preparation of wines the grapes are pressed either by their own weight, by treading or by putting them through wine presses. The grape juice, or "must," is poured into wooden vats where it is allowed to ferment under the influence of the yeast cells present on the skins of the grapes. The fermentation stops when the alcohol reaches a maximum of about 16% because at this concentration the alcohol poisons the yeast cells. After fermentation, the wine is purified and casked.

For red wines the skins of the grapes are fermented along with the juice. For white wines the skins are removed before fermentation. Natural wines, e.g., claret, contain only as much alcohol as has been produced by fermentation from the sugar of the grape juice. Fortified wines, such as port, sherry and Madeira, have spirit added to them. Champagne is a sparkling wine because it has been allowed to undergo a secondary fermentation in the bottle and is thus aerated with carbon dioxide. Cider and perry are prepared in a similar way to wines from apples and pears respectively. Home-made wines can be made by adding yeast to a syrup of fruit juice and sugar. The usual home-made wines are those of dandelion, damson, cherry, elderberry and blackberry. Natural wines contain roughly 10% alcohol and fortified wines some 20%.

Recent years have seen a revival of interest in the making of mead, a fermented drink in which honey is an important ingredient.

SPIRITS AND LIQUEURS

Spirits are fermented liquids which have been distilled to increase the concentration of the alcohol and other volatile substances. Whisky is distilled from fermented barley malt mash or a fermented mash of barley, rye, maize and malt. Rum is distilled from fermented molasses or the fermented juice of sugar cane. Genuine brandy is distilled wine. Gin is distilled from a fermented mash of rye and malt afterwards flavoured with juniper berries. Liqueurs are spirits sweetened with cane sugar and flavoured with herbs and essences. Spirits contain about 40% alcohol and liqueurs about the same amount of alcohol with about 30% sugar in addition.

USES OF ALCOHOLIC BEVERAGES

The use of alcoholic beverages has always been a much disputed question but we are not concerned here with the moral or economic aspects.

The use of alcohol as a medicine has greatly decreased in recent years. Other drugs can produce the same results without harmful after effects. Alcohol is a narcotic drug and never a stimulant. It has a sedative action on different parts of the central nervous system and thus deadens pain and relieves worry and anxiety.

Alcohol is an energy food of limited value. It is more rapidly absorbed than any other food since it can pass directly through the walls of the stomach and intestines into the blood stream, but it is not quickly oxidised.

Alcohol dilates the surface bloodvessels and so causes an extra flow of blood to the skin. This gives an illusory feeling of warmth but this is only temporary and is followed by an increased loss of heat so the final result is a chilling and not a warming.

Alcohol is quite unable to cure any disease, infectious or otherwise, or increase bodily strength, as is often supposed.

13 Flavouring and Colouring Materials

Foods are frequently made more attractive in taste, flavour and appearance by the addition of a wide range of spices, herbs, condiments, flavouring and colouring agents. There is no doubt that the taste, flavour and appearance of foods have considerable influence upon appetite and the flow of digestive juices and consequently upon digestion. In this sense, the use of flavouring and colouring materials, in moderation, is beneficial.

Particular flavourings are associated with particular foods, e.g., mustard with roast beef, mint sauce with lamb, sage and onion with pork and fowl, lemon juice with fillets of fish, and vinegar with crab and oysters. Pepper and salt have a universal application in the kitchen and at the dining table. Sauces, chutneys and salad creams have some food value but do not, of course, play a very significant role in the diet because of the small quantities normally eaten. Sauces and chutneys contain fruit, vinegar and sugar, while salad creams contain fat, vinegar and egg yolk. Mint and parsley contain vitamin C but, again, not sufficient is eaten to add much to the diet. Onions and leeks are also foods as well as flavourings.

The aroma and taste of flowers, fruits, leaves and other parts of plants used as flavouring agents are due mainly to the essential oils they contain. These essential oils must be distinguished from mineral oils, such as paraffin, on the one hand, and food oils, such as olive oil, on the other. Generally, essential oils are colourless liquids when pure and have strong odours and tastes. They are very volatile and some of them are easily destroyed by exposure to air. Consequently, extracts of essential oils used as flavourings should be kept in well-stoppered bottles to prevent loss by evaporation and loss of flavour by oxidation. Essential oils are not usually soluble in water but dissolve easily in alcohol. Flavouring essences or extracts are solutions of essential oils in alcohol.

Spices and condiments are now much less important and used in much smaller quantities than in mediaeval times or even fifty

K

years ago. In the Middle Ages pastures were poor and root crops for the winter feeding of farm animals unknown. With the approach of winter the greater part of the herd had to be slaughtered and the only method of preservation was by salting. By the end of the winter the meat was tough and unpalatable or even repulsive because of decay. The use of large quantities of spices, herbs and condiments was essential to give some variety to the monotonous salty flavour or to hide the unpleasant taste and flavour of half-rotten meat. Even fifty years ago the housewife's equipment included a comprehensive range of spices. Spices were the grocer's most important wares. In France the grocer is still called "l'épicier"—the spice dealer. Not only were spices and herbs used as flavourings but also as ingredients of medicines, salves and ointments. Nowadays, instead of being necessities spices and herbs have become merely pleasant adjuncts to foods.

SPICES

Spices were probably first brought to Europe by Arab merchants and Arabia was regarded as the home of spices although, in actual fact, most of them came from Southern India and the Moluccas, or Spice Islands. During the Middle Ages most of the spice trade was carried out by the Venetians and the glories of Venice and its empire of the seas were built upon it. By the end of the fifteenth century the trade had passed to the Portuguese. It is sometimes suggested that the voyages of Vasco da Gama and Columbus were originally planned to discover new routes to the spice islands of the East. From the Portuguese the spice trade passed to the Dutch and their East Indies Empire. Later most of the tropical and subtropical spice-producing countries and islands, such as India, Sri Lanka, Jamaica, East and West Africa, Tanzania and Grenada were, for a time, all in the British Commonwealth.

Spices can be classified according to the parts of plants from which they are derived, e.g.:

(a) *Fruit Spices*
Pepper, capsicums, chillies, paprika, pimento, vanilla.

(b) *Seed Spices*
Mustard, mace, nutmeg, cardamom, fenugreek, caraway and coriander.

(c) *Flower Spices*
Cloves, saffron, capers.

(d) *Bark Spices*
Cinnamon, cassia.
(e) *Root Spices*
Ginger, turmeric.

Fruit Spices
Pepper is the most important of the spices and has the widest use. Whole black pepper is the unripe fruit or berry of a tropical perennial creeper or vine. White pepper is a product of the same plant with the seeds in a riper state and with the outside skin removed. Peppers are grown chiefly in the Isle of Banka and Java. Singapore and Sarawak are the chief places from which pepper is exported.

The bulk of domestic pepper is in the form of ground pepper. For table use, white pepper is usually preferred because of its appearance when sprinkled on food but for kitchen use black pepper has the advantage in aroma and pungency. The aroma and pungency of pepper are due to an essential oil which stimulates the flow of saliva and gastric juice.

Capsicums and chillies are the fruits of various tropical perennials. The fruits vary considerably in shape, size, colour and taste. The large fruits are the capsicums and the small ones the chillies. Chillies are much the more pungent. Both types are widely grown in tropical countries. Capsicums are exported mainly from India and chillies from Japan and Nigeria. The main use of capsicums and chillies is in pickling spices.

Cayenne pepper is the name given to ground capsicums and chillies. Its colour varies from a bright red to a yellowish brown, according to the varieties and qualities of capsicums and chillies used in its preparation. It is not a substitute for ground black or white pepper. Its flavour is quite different. Because of its pungency, cayenne pepper is a common constituent of curry powders, chutneys, sauces, pickles and savouries.

Paprika or Hungarian pepper is the red pepper made from the dried ripe fruit of a capsicum grown in Hungary, Spain, U.S.A. and Chile. It has only a slight pungency and is mainly valuable as a colouring and garnishing in gravies, stews, hashes, ketchups and sauces.

Pimento or Allspice is the dried unripe fruit of a tropical evergreen myrtle grown in the West Indies. The berries are nearly globular in shape and of a light brown colour. The alternative name of allspice is derived from the supposed resemblance of its flavour to a mixture of cinnamon, nutmeg and cloves. It is also sometimes called Jamaica pepper. Pimento is much used, either whole or ground, in mixed spice, pickles, sauces, sausages and potted meats.

Seed Spices

Mustard is made by grinding the seeds of the black mustard and white mustard plants. In this country we use a mixture of the two types along with turmeric to give colour and wheat flour to absorb the essential oils and retard fermentation. White mustard seed is grown in East Anglia and is three times the size of the black seed but has less pungency and aroma. When mixed with cold water, vinegar or oil, the enzymes in the ground mustard flour produce the volatile mustard oil with its pungent smell and taste. The use of hot water or milk would destroy the enzymes and result in a mustard lacking in flavour. Mustard flour is used as a table condiment with cold meats. It assists digestion by promoting the flow of digestive juices. Whole mustard seeds are used in pickles and chutneys.

Mace and Nutmeg are both derived from the fruit of the nutmeg tree grown extensively in the East and West Indies. The fruit resembles an apricot. Mace is the dried red husk surrounding the kernel. The nutmeg is the kernel itself; both are used as flavourings.

Cardamoms are the small dark brown seeds of the cardamom plant grown in Sri Lanka, India, Java and Jamaica. The seeds are rich in an essential oil and are used for flavouring soups, sauces and cordials or "soft drinks."

Fenugreek consists of small yellowish-brown seeds of a plant grown chiefly in Morocco and Tunis. It is a common ingredient of curry powders to which it imparts colour, aroma and flavour.

Coriander is the globular seed of a plant grown extensively in India and Morocco. When ripe the seeds are very fragrant and have a pleasant, warm, pungent taste. They are important ingredients in curry powders, mixed spice and fancy breads and confectionery.

Caraway is the aromatic seed of a plant grown in Holland and other European countries. Caraway seeds are used in flavouring cakes and baked fruits.

Celery Seed is the seed of the celery plant grown in this country. It is useful as a flavouring when celery is out of season.

Flower Spices

Cloves are the dried unopened flower buds of a tropical evergreen tree grown chiefly in the Moluccas Islands, the Amboyna Islands, Tanzania and Madagascar. They are strongly aromatic, with a very characteristic odour and hot taste. Cloves are used in stews, steamed puddings, pickles, chutneys, and baked or stewed apples.

Saffron consists of the dried stigmas and tops of the styles of the saffron crocus which is grown chiefly in Spain. The town of Saffron Walden in Essex is supposed to have derived its name from the fact that the saffron crocus was grown there in large quantities in the sixteenth century. Saffron has a bright yellow colour, a very characteristic odour and a rather bitter taste. It is used in the saffron cakes popular in Cornwall and the West Country.

Capers are the flower buds of a tropical creeping shrub which are pickled in salt and vinegar and then dried. They are used in pickling spices and sauces.

Bark Spices

Cinnamon is the product of an evergreen aromatic laurel which grows wild and is cultivated in Sri Lanka. The Chinese, who discovered it when trading with Sri Lanka in the thirteenth century, found it was superior to their own cassia. The Portuguese occupied the island for the sake of its cinnamon after their discovery of the route via the Cape of Good Hope at the end of the fifteenth century. The Dutch captured the island in the seventeenth century and began the cultivation of the cinnamon tree. The island used to be part of the British Commonwealth.

The cultivated trees are kept as shrubs by severe pruning. After cutting the shoots, the twigs and leaves are removed and the bark slit down on both sides. The bark is then carefully removed, left for a few days to ferment and dry and finally cut into quills.

Cinnamon is used for flavouring cakes and puddings as well as pickles and chutneys.

Cassia, like cinnamon, is the product of an evergreen aromatic laurel. It is grown chiefly in China and is cheaper than cinnamon but inferior in flavour. Cassia is largely used in mixed spice.

Root Spices

Ginger was one of the earliest Oriental spices to be brought to Europe. It appears to have been used in China and India as a spice and medicine from the very earliest times. Its cultivation in Jamaica was started by the Spaniards in the sixteenth century. Jamaica still grows the finest ginger.

Ginger is prepared from the underground stem or rhizome of a tropical herbaceous perennial. The rhizomes are dug up, carefully peeled and dried. The dried rhizomes can be ground to a powder or preserved in syrup. Ginger is used by mineral water manufacturers and by the housewife as a flavouring.

Turmeric or Indian Saffron is obtained from the rhizome of a plant similar to the ginger plant. It is grown chiefly in India. The dried powdered rhizome is not very aromatic but, because of its rich yellow colour, is used to colour curry powder and mustard pickles. Its acrid taste makes it unsuitable for use in cakes.

Curry Powder is a mixture of ground spices such as coriander, turmeric, ginger, pepper, cardamoms, chillies, pimento, fenugreek and nutmeg.

HERBS

The sweet herbs used in the kitchen are the dried parts of plants—leaves, roots, fruits and seeds—which, because of the pungency and fragrance of their essential oils, give flavour to soups, stews, salads and so on.

Most of the herbs are native to the dry sunny soils of the Mediterranean countries. They were introduced to this country first by the Romans and later by the various orders of monks. Herb gardens were a characteristic feature of monasteries in mediaeval times. The only vegetables grown were onions and leeks and these were used as flavourings rather than as foods. Herbs, like the more pungent Oriental spices, were used to mask the flavour of the salted meat in stuffings and stews.

The herbs used included balm, basil, sage, marjoram, rosemary, mint, thyme, parsley, dill, fennel, angelica, aniseed, rue, borage, sweet bay, chervil, chive, garlic, horse-radish and tarragon. Those most commonly used today are parsley, mint, sage and thyme.

Parsley is grown largely for its leaves, which serve as garnishing and flavouring. It can be used fresh or dried and powdered.

Parsley, when fresh, is very rich in vitamin A and C and rich in riboflavine calcium and iron. Enough is eaten in parsley sauce to appreciably improve the diet.

Mint is made into sauce or jelly and eaten with lamb which it makes more digestible by stimulating the digestive glands. A few sprigs added to the water in which potatoes, peas or carrots are being boiled improve their flavour.

Sage leaves are used as flavouring and seasoning in soups and in stuffings with onion for ducks, geese and pork.

Thyme is the cultivated form of the wild thyme of the Mediterranean coast and is used in stuffings and salad dressings.

COMMON SALT

Although used in very large quantities as a condiment, salt is quite different in character from the spices and herbs. Unlike them, it is a mineral salt and is an essential food since it is a constituent of the blood. The hydrochloric acid of gastric juice is formed from it.

Most of the salt used in this country is obtained from Cheshire where it is pumped out of bore holes in the form of brine which is evaporated until the salt crystallises out. In hot countries salt is prepared by the evaporation of sea water in shallow ponds or salterns. In very cold countries the tide is trapped in shallow lagoons and allowed to freeze. The ice formed contains no salt and consequently the liquid below the ice contains an increased amount. This "concentrated" sea water is evaporated in pans over fires.

Even in this country during the Middle Ages salt was largely obtained by the evaporation of sea water run into shallow salterns. Traces of these may still be found in the neighbourhood of Portsmouth, Lymington and Poole. From the centres of this sea-salt industry and from the naturally occurring brine springs at Droitwich and Northwich, ancient tracks, the saltways, carried a considerable traffic in salt throughout the country. In those days, as we have seen, salt had a very extensive use as a preservative of meat, fowl and fish.

Salt is added to most food during its preparation or cooking. It is used as a preservative, either as dry salt or as brine. (See pp. 174, 175.) The addition of salt to the water in which fish or vegetables are cooked helps to prevent the loss of their natural mineral salts and so preserves their flavour. Salt is used in breadmaking as a flavouring and also to strengthen the gluten and moderate the fermentation. The addition of a small quantity of salt to egg white before whisking it helps to stabilise the foam.

Some brands of table salt have a little rice powder or sodium phosphate added to them to prevent impurities in the salt absorbing moisture from the air and so becoming damp or caking in lumps. Iodised table salts have small amounts of iodine compounds added to them. They are recommended for use in districts where the drinking water and vegetables are deficient in iodine and goitre is consequently prevalent. (See page 41.)

VINEGAR

Vinegar, or "sour wine," is formed when light alcoholic beverages such as weak wines, cider and ale are left exposed to the air. The alcohol they contain is oxidised to acetic acid by acetic acid bacteria. The alcoholic taste is changed to the sharp sour taste of vinegar. Strong alcoholic beverages such as port wine and whisky cannot be fermented to vinegar by these bacteria.

Genuine vinegars are made from poor quality wine, cider or malt liquor by fermentation with acetic acid bacteria. In this country, malt liquor is mainly used. The malt liquor is first fermented by yeast to convert the glucose of the malt into alcohol and then fermented by acetic acid bacteria to convert the alcohol into acetic acid and so produce malt vinegar.

Cheap artificial vinegars are made by diluting industrial acetic acid with water and adding a little caramel to colour it. Such vinegars have a harshness and pungency lacking in fermented vinegars.

The sharp sour flavour of vinegar makes it a useful condiment with fish, crabs, oysters and salads. The acetic acid of vinegar acts as a preservative in pickles and chutneys.

FLAVOURING ESSENCES OR EXTRACTS

Genuine fruit essences or extracts are solutions in alcohol of the essential oils and esters of fruits which flavour any confectionery in which they are used. With a few exceptions, such as vanilla, lemon, orange and almond, it is impossible to extract the distinctive flavours from fruits in sufficient quantity and of sufficient strength for flavouring purposes. For this reason the majority of fruit essences are artificial products prepared by mixing artificial essential oils and esters with alcohol. The aroma and flavour of such artificial essences are seldom as delicate or as fragrant as the natural product they attempt to imitate. Occasionally, an artificial essence contains only a single substance dissolved in alcohol, e.g., amyl acetate (pear drops), but more usually several substances are used in varying proportions before close approximation to the natural product is achieved.

In certain cases, better results are obtained by using the actual source of the flavouring rather than the essence. Thus finely cut orange and lemon peels mixed in cakes gives a flavour superior to that obtained with the essences.

Vanilla Essence

The flavour of vanilla is due to a substance called vanillin. The vanilla pods from which the vanillin is extracted are the fruits of a tropical climbing orchid. The pods or beans, which are greenish-yellow in colour when gathered before they are fully ripe, are allowed to ferment. The flavouring material, vanillin, is formed in the beans and appears as white crystals on the outside of the beans. After drying in the sun, the beans have a dark brown wrinkled surface and a waxy feel. They are about 20 cm long and about 6 mm thick in the middle. They are tied into bundles for export.

The pods may be crushed to a powder and mixed with nine times their weight of castor sugar and used in this dry form, or the pods may be broken into small pieces and steeped in alcohol for several months to form vanilla essence.

Artificial vanilla essence is prepared by dissolving synthetic vanillin in alcohol. It is inferior to the natural product.

Lemon and Orange Essences

The essential oils of these two citrus fruits occur in small glands in the rinds from which they are extracted by pressure. On the large scale, screw presses are used, but the finest quality oils are produced by hand. One hand method is the sponge and bowl process in which the peel is cut into halves and the oil expressed by turning them inside out and then wiping off the oil with a sponge and squeezing the sponge in a bowl. In another hand process the rind is rotated rapidly in a round metal bowl studded with sharp spikes which burst the glands containing the oil. The extracted oil collects in a receptacle at the bottom of the bowl.

These oils are produced mainly in Sicily and Southern Italy and, more recently, in California. They are pale yellow in colour with characteristic aromas and bitter aromatic tastes. The extracts or essences are prepared by diluting the oils with alcohol.

Almond Essence

There are two types of almonds—sweet almonds and bitter almonds. Sweet almonds are used, either whole or ground, for marzipan, almond paste and dessert. It is the bitter almond whose kernel is used for the extraction of almond oil. The essential oil of bitter almonds is benzaldehyde and artificial almond essence is simply a solution of artificial benzaldehyde in alcohol.

Before concluding this section we ought to point out that although sugar is a valuable energy food and is commonly regarded as such, it is, nevertheless, the most widely used of all flavouring agents. Like the others, when used in moderation, it stimulates the appetite and the flow of digestive juices.

COLOURING MATERIALS

Not only are foods made more palatable to the taste by the use of flavouring materials but their appearance is sometimes made more pleasing to the eye by the addition of colouring materials. Some of the colours used are natural animal or vegetable products such as caramel, cochineal, turmeric, annatto and saffron. Others are artificial coal tar dyes or inorganic pigments such as are used in textile dyeing. Of the three types, the artificial coal tar dyes, on account of their very wide range in colour, are the most important.

Unfortunately, many coal tar dyes and inorganic pigments are toxic and some, if consumed, even in very small quantities, over a long period, may produce cancer. According to the Colouring Matter in Food Regulations, 1957, apart from natural vegetable products, only certain inorganic pigments believed to be innocuous and various artificial dyes also thought to be harmless, are permitted in foods.

Cochineal or Carmine

Cochineal is prepared from the female insect (*coccina*) which feeds upon a variety of cactus native to Mexico and Peru and cultivated in Guatemala and the Canary Islands. The female insects are collected and killed by dropping them into hot water and then dried in the sun. Alternatively, the insects may be placed in bags and dried in stoves without previously killing in hot water. The essential colouring matter in cochineal is carminic acid.

Annatto

Annatto is prepared from the fermented seeds of a tropical plant cultivated in the West Indies and Sri Lanka. The dye is sold as an orange paste and is used in colouring butter, margarine and cheese. *Turmeric* and *Saffron* which are used as both flavouring and colouring materials have already been described.

14 Raising Agents

Raising agents are substances that are introduced into foods so as to make them lighter. However, it must be remembered that the food must remain in its puffed-up state, and so one relies on the stretching and setting powers of gluten, egg and gelatine; otherwise the food will only remain "puffed up" for a short time.

The most natural raising agents are air and steam; yeast can be used to introduce gas into a mixture, or chemicals can be used singly or combined together to produce gas.

AIR

Air is introduced into a mixture by mechanical means, for example the sieving of flour, the beating of egg, margarine and sugar in a cake mixture, and the kneading of a bread or scone mixture.

STEAM

Most foods contain some water, and when the water is heated it is transformed into steam. This steam can lift the mixture as effectively as any other gas.

YEAST

(See also page 156.) Yeast is a single-celled plant; it feeds on carbohydrates, converting starch to maltose and absorbing and using all forms of sugar as a source of energy.

If there is a plentiful supply of air, yeast is able to use the sugar in the normal way, oxidising the sugar to carbon dioxide and water. As a result of this oxidation, 1 gramme of sugar liberates 3·75 kcals.

glucose + oxygen = carbon dioxide + water + free energy

$$C_6H_{12}O_6 + 6O_2 = 6CO_2 + 6H_2O$$

This is the normal process of respiration and is called *aerobic respiration.* Yeast is, also, capable of getting energy from sugar without using oxygen. This process is called *anaerobic respiration.* The glucose is broken down to carbon dioxide and alcohol, and energy is liberated. Because the sugar is not fully broken down, less energy is liberated.

glucose = carbon dioxide + alcohol

$$C_6H_{12}O_6 = 2CO_2 + 2C_2H_5OH$$

After a while the quantity of alcohol increases and eventually becomes so great that it inactivates the yeast.

As can be seen from the molecular formulae above, when yeast is working aerobically six parts of carbon dioxide are produced for every one part of glucose, whereas in anaerobic respiration it produces only two parts of carbon dioxide to every part of glucose. Thus for aerating purposes, anaerobic respiration is far less efficient than aerobic respiration.

In both aerobic and anaerobic respiration the temperature will affect the rate of activity of the yeast. The activity decreases with decreasing temperature, but if heated too much the yeast will be damaged. Approximately blood heat (36·9° C) is the best temperature.

When using yeast to make a dough mixture, the yeast is first mixed with milk, and sugar is added. This is to start the yeast off, as it metabolises sugar more easily than the starch of flour (which must first be converted to maltose). The milk is warmed to blood heat as the yeast is at its maximum rate of activity at that temperature.

After about ten minutes the yeast is then added to the warm flour and the mixture is thoroughly kneaded. The main reason for this is to stretch the gluten, but it also mixes the yeast thoroughly with the flour and encloses air within the mixture.

When the dough is left in a warm place to rise the yeast will utilise any remaining sugar and air respiring aerobically, but this will be followed by utilisation of flour and anaerobic respiration, and as the yeast grows so it will multiply. The gases given off are trapped within the mixture and lift it.

The risen dough is now taken and "knocked back." This knock-back drives out some of the gas, splits up the remainder evenly and, as important, spreads the now much increased yeast evenly throughout the mixture, putting it into contact with more food. The dough is now left to rise again before cooking, and the yeast again gives off carbon dioxide and alcohol. The risen dough is then cooked.

During cooking, the yeast is killed, the alcohol and some water evaporate. All the gases expand, lifting the dough still further, and as they are driven off, so the mixture sets in its risen state.

CHEMICAL RAISING AGENTS

The simplest chemical raising agent is sodium bicarbonate ("bicarb"). When it is heated it gives off carbon dioxide.

$$\text{sodium bicarbonate} \xrightarrow{\text{heated}} \text{sodium carbonate} + \text{carbon dioxide} + \text{water}$$

$$2Na(HCO_3) = Na_2CO_3 + CO_2 + H_2O$$

As can be seen from the chemical equation, two parts of sodium bicarbonate give off one part of carbon dioxide and sodium carbonate is left as a residue. This residue browns the flour and gives a characteristic taste to the food; the use of bicarbonate of soda on its own is limited by these factors.

If sodium bicarbonate is used with an acid, a reaction will take place; all the carbon dioxide will be liberated and the sodium will form the salt of the acid. Thus with acetic acid (vinegar) the resulting salt is sodium acetate, with lemon juice, which contains citric acid, it is sodium citrate, and so on. The stronger the acid the faster the reaction will take place.

$$\text{sodium bicarbonate} + \text{acetic acid} \rightarrow \text{sodium acetate} + \text{carbon dioxide} + \text{water}$$

$$Na(HCO_3) + CH_3COOH = CH_3COONa + CO_2 + H_2O$$

As can be seen from the above equation, in this reaction (contrast with first equation above) one part of sodium bicarbonate liberates one part of carbon dioxide. There is also the advantage that an approximately neutral salt is formed which will not discolour the flour or taste strongly.

The disadvantage of these agents is that once the acid is mixed with the sodium bicarbonate the reaction proceeds extremely quickly. Much of the gas is given off before the food has had time to be cooked and the gas therefore escapes from the food before it is set in its raised position. To minimise this effect a weak acid in a powder form can be used, e.g., tartaric acid.

sodium bicarbonate + tartaric acid → sodium tartrate + carbon dioxide + water

$$2Na(HCO_3) + \begin{array}{l} CHOH.COOH \\ | \\ CHOH.COOH \end{array} = \begin{array}{l} CHOH.COONa \\ | \\ CHOH.COONa \end{array} + 2CO_2 + 2H_2O$$

Weaker still, an acid salt can be used—for instance, cream of tartar or potassium acid tartrate. This salt does not dissolve in cold liquid and so the reaction does not start until the mixture is heated.

potassium hydrogen tartrate + sodium bicarbonate → sodium potassium tartrate + carbon dioxide + water

$$\begin{array}{l} CHOH.COOH \\ | \\ CHOH.COOK \end{array} + Na(HCO_3) = \begin{array}{l} CHOH.COONa \\ | \\ CHOH.COOK \end{array} + CO_2 + H_2O$$

Sometimes commercial baking powders use calcium hydrogen phosphate as the acid salt.

sodium bicarbonate + calcium hydrogen phosphate → Calcium disodium dihydrogen phosphate + carbon dioxide + water

$$2Na(HCO_3) + CaH_4(PO_4)_2 = CaNa_2H_2(PO_4)_2 + 2CO_2 + 2H_2O$$

But though calcium hydrogen phosphate is cheap it also dissolves in cold water, and so if the powder gets damp the reaction will start.

Because of this acid sodium pyrophosphate is usually preferred as it will not react with sodium bicarbonate until the mixture is heated.

sodium bicarbonate + disodium dihydrogen phosphate → disodium hydrogen phosphate + carbon dioxide + water

$$2Na(HCO_3) + Na_2H_2P_2O_7 = 2Na_2HPO_4 + 2CO_2 + H_2O$$

Commercial baking powders frequently contain a third ingredient as a "filler." This is usually some form of starch such as rice flour or cornflour which will help to keep the baking powder dry by absorbing any small amounts of moisture with which it may come into contact.

The use of chemical raising agents

The choice of raising agents and the amount that is needed will depend on various factors.

1. Sometimes the raising action is required to take place very quickly; for instance, when making honeycomb toffee, when the

raising agent is introduced just as the sugar has reached its setting point. In such a case the use of a free acid with the bicarbonate is advisable.

2. Sometimes the taste or colouring effects of the raising agent residue are necessary to the finished dish—for instance in soda bread or soda scones, where a slight sodium carbonate residue is needed.

3. Sometimes some of the ingredients are themselves acid, and allowance for this is needed in the choice of raising agents—for instance, lemon juice or sour milk can be used as flavourings and will provide the necessary acid to liberate all the carbon dioxide from the sodium bicarbonate.

4. The amount of raising agents used must be balanced against the weights of the other ingredients, and the strength of the supporting ingredients. For instance, in a mixture in which there are equal quantities of egg, flour, fat and sugar, the air entrapped by beating the fat and sugar and whisking the egg is sufficient to hold up the mixture. However, if one reduces the relative quantity of egg, then a chemical raising agent is added to help to aerate the mixture.

5. The amount of raising agent used is also affected by what sort of structure is wanted in the final product:— for instance, is the open texture of a sponge cake required? or the closer texture of a fruit cake?

PART THREE

15 The Preservation of Foods

No food will keep indefinitely in its natural form. All natural foods are "alive" and, like all other living materials, are subject to processes of deterioration and decay. These gradual changes in fresh foods are due partly to chemical changes in the living protoplasm of the food itself, usually catalysed by the cell enzymes, and partly to changes caused by minute organisms which get into the foods from outside.

Meat, fish and eggs go putrid, fats go rancid, milk goes sour, fruits go mouldy or ferment, vegetables wilt and rot, cereals go musty or germinate, because of the action of enzymes. All natural foods are slowly and continually changing in character and composition. Their appearance, smell, flavour and food value are gradually being altered. The preservation of food consists in the stopping or slowing down of these changes.

These changes are not always harmful or undesirable. We have seen that cream is "ripened" before it is churned into butter, that cheese is allowed to "ripen" to develop flavour, and that meat is "hung" to make it more digestible. But there comes a stage in the decay of most foods when they become obnoxious or harmful and even, in some cases, poisonous.

It is obviously desirable to eat fresh foods whenever we can but this is not always possible. Such a large proportion of the world's population lives in large towns and cities away from farms and gardens that food has to be transported great distances and kept in good condition for long periods. Some countries produce more food than they can consume themselves while every country produces surpluses of such foods as fruits, vegetables and eggs at certain seasons of the year. Modern civilisation could not exist without the use of preserved foods. But for the use of methods of preservation much of the world's food would be wasted and our diets would be much less varied than they are. Preserved foods usually require less preparation and less cooking than raw fresh

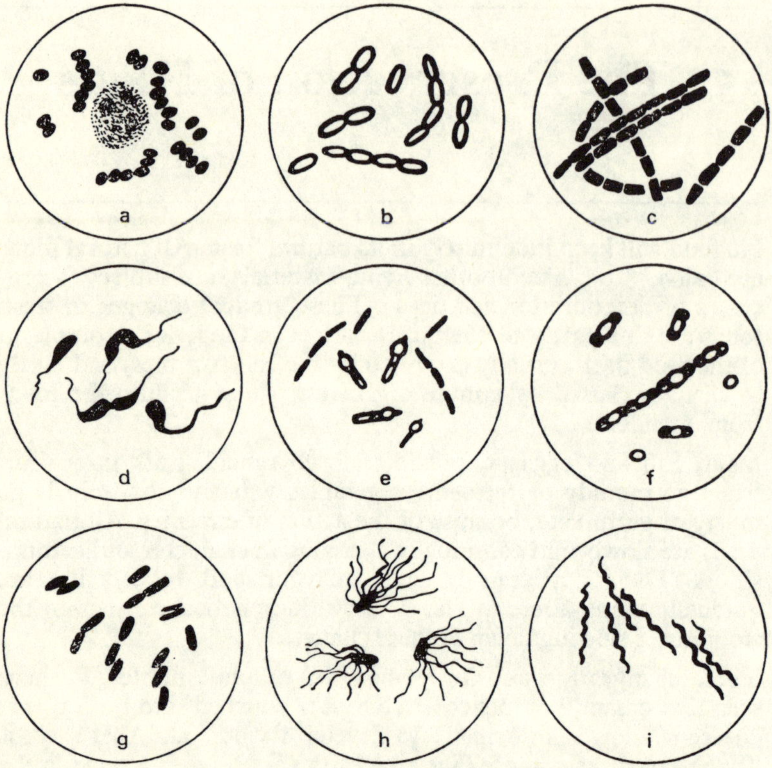

Bacteria. (a) Streptococci from pus (showing a blood corpuscle); (b) *Pneumococcus* (pneumonia); (c) *Bacillus anthracis* (anthrax), showing bacilli in chains; (d) cholera spirillum showing flagellate cells; (e) *Clostridium tetani* (tetanus) showing cells with and without spores; (f) *Bacillus anthracis* showing the formation of a single spore inside each bacterial cell; (g) (h) *Bacillus typhosus* (typhoid) with and without flagella; (i) *Spirochaeta pallida*—a protozoon.

foods and so have the merit of convenience. Their flavours are frequently altered but there is little loss of food value except for some loss of vitamins, particularly ascorbic acid and the B vitamins. Provided this is realised and fresh foods eaten to make up for this loss there is no harm in the increased use of preserved foods.

CHEMICAL CHANGES HELPED BY ENZYMES

Enzymes are substances present within all cells which speed up chemical reactions but remain unchanged themselves at the end of the reaction. Most enzymes can only work if water is present and there is not too high a concentration of acid, alkali, sugar or salt. Low temperatures slow down reaction rates and high temperatures destroy the enzymes.

MICRO-ORGANISMS CAUSING CHEMICAL CHANGES

The minute living organisms which attack foods are simple forms of plant life. They are of three types: bacteria, yeasts and moulds. To understand how food is preserved we must know something about the needs and habits of these organisms.

Bacteria

Bacteria are minute organisms consisting of single cells of great diversity of shape. Each cell contains a nucleus which is enclosed within the protoplasm of the cell, and they vary in size between $\frac{1}{1000}$ mm and $\frac{3}{1000}$ mm (1–3 microns) and vary in shape. Some possess long or short flagella (hair-like processes) which they can use to move around with.

Under suitable conditions bacteria can multiply very rapidly indeed, dividing in half about every twenty minutes. This means that in such conditions a very small number of bacteria can soon develop into a large population.

Under certain conditions some bacteria can enclose the essential part of the cell within a resistant wall and thus form a very resistant cell called a spore. The spores can withstand degrees of drying, heat, and cold which would destroy the normal cell.

Bacteria require suitable food, ample moisture, warmth, and some require oxygen. The food that bacteria need varies enormously; some bacteria can live on fuel oils, others live in the soil, in our intestines and so on, but the ones we are concerned with in this chapter can use our food as their own.

Bacteria vary in the amount of heat that they prefer and fall roughly into three groups: those that like warmth and which flourish at temperatures of 42–75° C; those that like moderate temperatures between 10–20° C (about average room temperature) and those which can grow at temperatures as low as 0° C, which is well below that of a household refrigerator.

Bacteria do not all need oxygen; some can live without it if necessary and others actually require anaerobic conditions.

How to stop the growth of bacteria

Acids, strong solutions of sugar, or salt can prevent the growth of most bacteria, and they cannot develop without water. Low temperatures slow the growth of bacteria, and if the temperature is sufficiently low it will stop their growth completely. However, once warmer conditions return the bacteria will become active again, and in fact it has been found that they are more active after being chilled than they were before. High temperatures will destroy bacteria but some bacteria are much more susceptible than others and the spores of some bacteria can resist boiling for many hours.

YEASTS

Like bacteria, these are small single-celled organisms. They are oval in shape and measure about 7 microns across, which is much bigger than most bacteria. The cells consist of protoplasm with a denser part in the middle called the nucleus. They multiply by the process of budding. A small bud appears on the side of the yeast

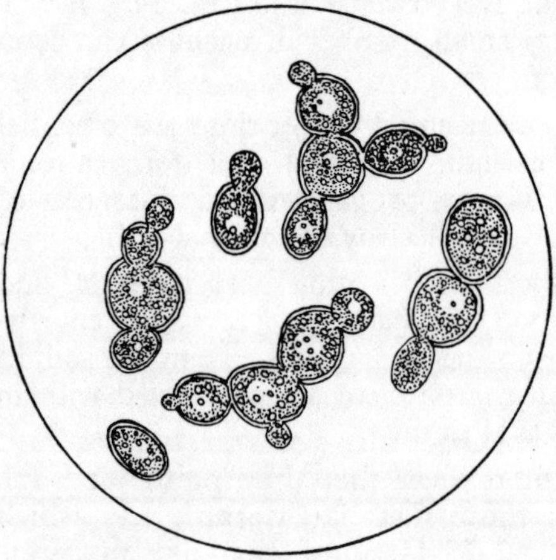

Yeast cells and budding.

cell, grows larger and eventually splits off as an independent yeast cell. Yeast cells can form resistant spores under unfavourable conditions in a similar way to bacteria.

Yeasts need less moisture than bacteria and can tolerate a greater degree of acidity and a higher concentration of sugar. They flourish in dilute sugar solutions and ferment sugar syrups, jam and fruit juices. Heat and cold affect yeasts in the same way as they affect bacteria.

MOULDS

Moulds are simple plants consisting of a network of branching threads which spread in all directions through the food. The threads are known as hyphae and the tangled mass as a mycelium. Here and there the hyphae develop stalks, known as filaments, which rise above the food and develop thousands of minute spores corresponding to the seeds of higher forms of plant life. In the

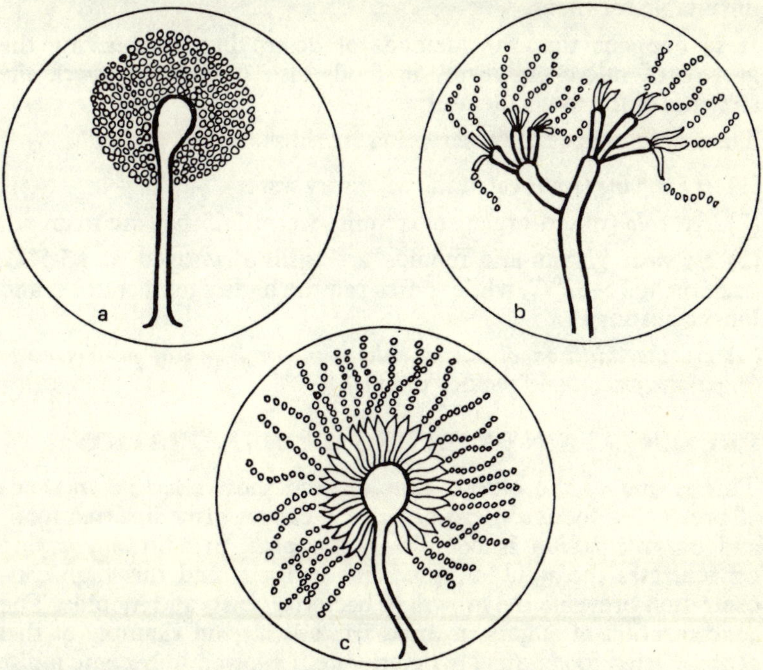

Moulds: (a) Mucor, (b) Penicillium, (c) Aspergillus.

group of moulds known as *Penicillium*, the spores are developed in chains from the tips of the branched hyphae. In the genus *Aspergillus* the spores are developed in chains which radiate from the swollen tip of a hypha. In the genus *Mucor*, a large number of spores are produced in a spore case which is developed at the tip of a hypha. By means of spores, moulds are spread over the food or are carried in the dust of the air to other foods.

Moulds require less moisture than either bacteria or yeasts and are not as much affected by acids, sugar and salt.

Thus we see that, for their growth, bacteria, yeasts and moulds require moisture, suitable temperature, suitable food, and sometimes oxygen. They are affected by high concentrations of acids, sugar and salt. The various methods of preservation of foods consist in the destruction of the micro-organisms they contain, the removal of one or more of the conditions necessary for their growth, or the addition of sugar, salt or acids to make the foods unsuitable for them.

It so happens that the methods of destroying or checking the growth of micro-organisms in foods also destroy or check the enzymes of the foods themselves.

The chief methods of preservation are thus:

(1) *By drying* (removal of the necessary water).

(2) *By cold* (micro-organisms require warmth if they are to grow).

(3) *By heat* (yeasts and moulds are easily destroyed at 65·5° C, bacteria at 71–82° C, while spores require higher temperatures and longer heating).

(4) *By the addition of sugar, salt, acids or chemical preservatives* (e.g., jam, bacon and pickled onions).

PRESERVATION BY DRYING OR DEHYDRATION

This is one of the oldest, simplest and most effective methods of preserving foods. Micro-organisms cannot grow in dried foods and enzyme action is completely stopped. In addition, drying concentrates the soluble ingredients in foods and this high concentration prevents the growth of bacteria, yeasts and moulds. The concentration of sugars in dried fruits is a good example of this action. Dried foods quickly deteriorate if allowed to become moist again as drying does not destroy either the enzymes of the food itself or the harmful micro-organisms. As soon as water is added to the food the enzymes and micro-organisms will become active again.

There are various different methods of drying foods. The oldest type relies on the natural drying out of food exposed to the sun and air; this method needs a climate more predictable than that of Britain. The use of heat to drive off the water is now common; the actual method used will depend on the food itself and how finely divided it is (thus one method may be used for kippers, another for herrings intended for pastes). The latest method to be developed is called freeze drying.

DRYING BY THE USE OF HEAT

Solids may either be hung-up or spread on trays and a current of hot air passed over them, or they may be put on to perforated trays and have warm air blown through from below.

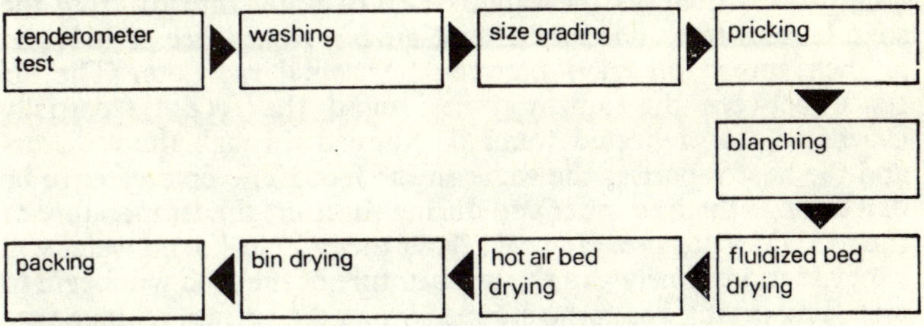

Processing of hot-air dried peas—flow-line diagram by courtesy of Unilever.

Stage 1. Pricking. The peas are pricked. This allows them to be quickly rehydrated.

Stage 2. Blanching. To destroy enzymes.

Stage 3. Fluidized hot-air beds. Hot air is blown through from below. The temperature of the air increases from 40°C in the first bed to 55°C in the seventh.

Stage 4. Hot-air beds. These rely on heat rather than on currents of air to drive off most of the remaining water.

Stage 5. Bin driers. The peas are finally kept in warm bins until the moisture content falls to between 5–7%.

Stage 6. Packaging. The peas must be packed in an atmosphere free from oxygen, usually in plastic-laminate.

Liquids may be dried by the *roller* or *spray* processes. In the roller process the food is allowed to fall on to hot revolving rollers. The water evaporates rapidly and leaves a thin film of powder on the rollers; this is automatically scraped off. In the spray process the liquid is pumped through fine jets and falls as a spray into a chamber through which hot air is circulated. The fine droplets of liquid quickly lose their water by evaporation and fall to the floor of the chamber as a fine powder.

The temperature of the hot air has to be carefully regulated in all these processes to avoid, so far as is possible, damaging the proteins and altering the taste. Inevitably, however, the hot air destroys any vitamin C present and some of the thiamine.

FREEZE-DRYING

Is carried out without the use of so much heat and, provided that the food is correctly packed afterwards, there is little loss of thiamine and ascorbic acid.

The process involves the vaporisation of water directly from the solid frozen state. The food is first quickly frozen (see p. 164) and is then spread on trays between horizontal radiators. The air space between the radiators, i.e. round the food, is partially evacuated, super-heated water is pumped through the radiators and the heat vaporises the water in the food. The first water to be driven off is the free water and during this time the temperature of the food does not rise. However, later the protein-bound water will vaporise more slowly and the temperature of the food will begin to rise. The drying has to be stopped when the surface temperature of the food rises to beyond 40°C in animal food and 60°C in plant food to avoid damaging the tissues. Between $1\frac{1}{2}$–3% moisture is left and the food itself, which will retain much of its original structure, is very friable. The vacuum in the drying machines is broken by flushing the machine with inert gases, and the food is packed in an atmosphere of nitrogen either in plastic-lined tins or in plastic and foil packets. The nitrogen replaces all air and as it is inert will not react with the contents. Were air present oxidation would occur.

Accelerated freeze-drying (a.f.d.) is a method of speeding up the drying time and was developed by the Ministry of Agriculture. It involves placing expanded metal sheets below and above the food in the drying cabinets. The time taken for the food to dry can be cut by almost half, but the food must be of absolutely uniform size and able to withstand the weight of the expanded metal sheets.

Correct packaging of freeze-dried food is important, as air, light and moisture must be excluded.

Meat

Dried meat is not much used in this country but beef has been dried by the natives of North America, South America and South Africa for centuries, where it is known respectively as pemmican, charqui and biltong. Dried beef has been used in recent times by Polar explorers and by soldiers as part of their "iron ration." Such meat not only keeps well but occupies very little space compared with fresh meat or meat preserved by other methods.

The meat is sliced and cooked until brown in the minimum amount of water. It is then minced and spread on trays and dried in a current of warm air. Finally, it is packed in airtight tins with nitrogen in place of air to prevent oxidation of the fat. Except for some loss of vitamin B_1 (thiamine) its nutritive value is similar to that of fresh beef.

Meat can also be freeze-dried.

Fish

Fish is still sun-dried, as it has been for centuries, in the Scandinavian countries, Canada, Newfoundland, India and all round the Mediterranean coasts. In this country, fish is roller dried like milk and eggs. Alternatively, it is filleted, minced and cooked for thirty minutes, then spread on trays and dehydrated in a current of warm air. Herrings are the fish most frequently dried here because, although the herring fishing season only lasts twenty weeks, such vast quantities are caught they cannot all be eaten fresh. The dehydrated herring is in the form of crumbly grey-brown pellets which can be reconstituted with milk, water, or water and vinegar for use in fish cakes and sandwich fillings.

Fish can also be freeze-dried.

Eggs

Liquid eggs can be dried by the roller process or the spray process. Precautions must be taken to prevent the coagulation of the proteins by keeping the temperature below coagulation point, otherwise the dried egg will not reconstitute properly when mixed with water. Even then there is some denaturing of the proteins, and dried eggs are not as good aerating agents as the same amount of fresh eggs. The addition of sugar to the liquid egg before drying gives the reconstituted egg improved aerating qualities. Except for some loss of thiamine there is little alteration of food value. Dried egg keeps well, particularly if sealed in airtight containers with nitrogen in place of air to prevent oxidation of the fat. It is easily transported and convenient in use. Dried egg has occasionally been found to contain Salmonella bacteria, and for this reason it is particularly important not to reconstitute the egg until just before you are ready to use it.

Milk

Milk can be dried by the roller or spray processes. Spray dried milk is probably the more successful of the two.

Fruits

Fruits have been dried from time immemorial and are, at the present time, the most popular of all dried foods. The old method, which is still used in hot countries, is to dry the fruit in the sun on fibre mats spread out on the ground. Drying on a commercial scale is now usually carried out by means of a current of warm air. On the small scale, in the home, fruits may be dried by placing them in a moderately warm oven on wire trays or wooden frames covered with muslin or cheese cloth.

Currants, sultanas and raisins are produced from special varieties of grapes grown for the purpose. Apples and pears are peeled, cored and cut into discs before drying. Apricots have their stones removed. Prunes are dried plums.

Because of the concentration of their sugars due to the removal of water, dried fruits such as currants, sultanas, raisins, dates and figs are valuable energy foods. Dried apples, pears, apricots and prunes are reconstituted by soaking in water before cooking and then resemble the original fresh fruits in flavour and food value except for the loss of ascorbic acid, some vitamin A and some thiamine.

Vegetables

Green leafy vegetables, such as cabbage, are first shredded and then "blanched" by dipping them into water containing sulphite (sulphur dioxide) and then scalding them in steam. This treatment destroys the enzymes which decompose ascorbic acid and also helps to prevent the cabbage becoming discoloured during dehydration. If this is not done there is considerable loss of ascorbic acid and much discolouration. The cabbage is then spread on trays and quickly dried at 95°C until it contains only 5% water. It is packed in sealed cans to prevent absorption of moisture from the air and if it is to be stored for a long time should have the air in the tin replaced by nitrogen.

Carrots are dehydrated in a similar way. There is some loss of carotene. As they will develop a smell of violets, due to oxidation of carotene, if exposed to the air for any length of time they must be packed in sealed tins filled with nitrogen.

Potatoes can be sliced, "blanched" and dried in the same way as cabbage and carrots and it is claimed that 50% of the original ascorbic acid is retained. Another method is to cook and mash the potatoes before drying. The dried powder is granulated and consists of unbroken starch cells which reconstitute with water to give an excellent mash. If the starch cells were burst, then a sticky paste would be formed with water.

Herbs can be preserved by washing, tying in bundles, covering with a piece of muslin to keep out dust and hanging up to dry. Those with large leaves may have the leaves plucked from the stalks, blanched in boiling water and dried in a cool oven until crisp. They may then be crushed to a powder and stored in tins or sealed jars.

Vegetables can be freeze-dried as already described.

Cereals and Pulses

Cereals and pulses are already dried by nature. They are dried plants in miniature with a dried food supply which they can only convert into soluble forms when they obtain the necessary water and begin to germinate. The preservation of cereals and pulses, and the meals and flours made from them, is merely a matter of keeping them dry.

PRESERVATION BY COLD

Although it has been known for a long time that the deterioration of foods can be delayed by low temperatures, it is only within the last seventy years or so that widespread use of this principle has been possible following the invention of the refrigerator. Refrigeration is applied to foods either to chill them or actually to freeze them, e.g., mutton carcases. In chilling, the food is kept at a temperature just above freezing point and is used with foods which do not recover their natural state after thawing, e.g., beef carcases.

It is important to realise that foods are made up of living cells, that every living cell contains a great deal of water and that dissolved in this water are many organisms and inorganic substances such as salts, sugars and acids as well as colloidal suspensions of proteins. Because of this high water content, most foods freeze solidly at temperatures about $-5°$C. If this freezing takes place slowly, as it does with large carcases of meat, the ice crystals formed are large enough to rupture the cell walls and to generally break down the texture. On thawing out, much of the liquid drains away, taking with it part of the minerals and vitamins which give the food its particular character. If the freezing can be done very rapidly, e.g., $-33°$C, the ice crystals formed in the cells are so small as not to damage the cellular structure, and the food returns to practically its original condition on thawing. This is the principle underlying the preparation of "quick-frozen" or "frosted" foods which are becoming increasingly popular. Small quantities of vegetables, fruit, fish and meat can be very successfully dealt with in this way. Peas, beans, strawberries, blackcurrants, cod, plaice, lamb cutlets and beef steaks are eminently suitable for this treatment.

Commercially there are two main methods of quick-freezing food. One is to put the food between the hollow plates which are filled with a refrigerant which is pumped round. This method is called the *plate* or *multi-plate* method, and is used for fish and meat as they take a relatively longer time to freeze than fruit and vegetables. The second method is called the *tunnel* method and is mainly used for fruit and vegetables. In this method the food is put on to a moving belt and carried past a current of cold air. There is a third method in which the food is actually immersed in liquid refrigerant but as this method is rather costly it is not used extensively.

In the home the food is frozen by putting it into the freezer section of the deep-freeze cabinet. Vegetables are first prepared, then blanched in boiling water to destroy the enzymes and are then

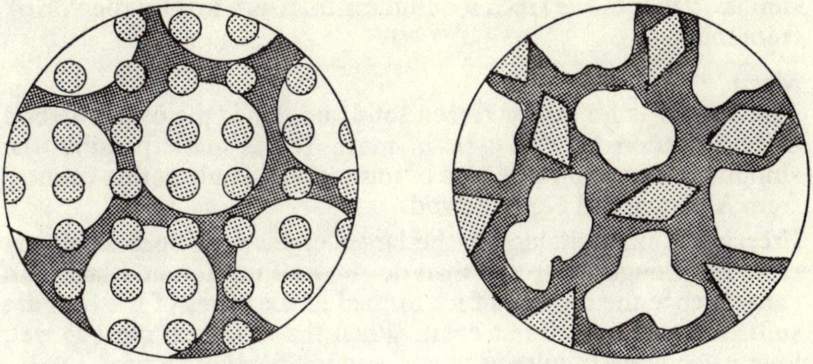

Diagrams illustrating the effects of (a) quick freezing and (b) slow freezing on the cellular structure of foodstuffs. By courtesy of Unilever.

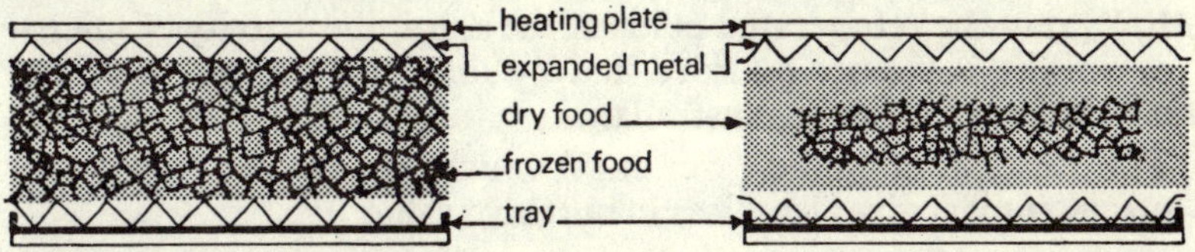

The position of the heating plates at the start of the drying cycle in accelerated freeze-drying (left) and part of the way through the cycle. By courtesy of Unilever.

packed in polythene bags before putting them into the freezing cabinet. Fruit may either be blanched or simply packed in sugar in cardboard cartons or polythene bags.

Whole meals can now be purchased which have been cooked and then quick-frozen and vacuum sealed in transparent plastic or in foil packets. The housewife has only to heat the packet, before opening it and serving the meal.

Refrigeration is only a temporary method of preservation. Micro-organisms are not destroyed by subjecting them to low temperatures; their growth is merely checked.

If micro-organisms are chilled and then thawed there is a noticeable increase in their activity over and above that which would normally occur at that temperature.

The nutritional value of food preserved by chilling or freezing is similar to that of the fresh food unless there is a loss by the "drip" from meat.

Meat

Mutton and lamb can be frozen solid and this is the usual method of preservation for this type of meat. It has made possible the shipping of thousands of tons of mutton and lamb to this country from Australia and New Zealand.

Freezing is not suitable for the larger carcases of beef. Beef carcases take longer to freeze than do those of mutton and lamb. In consequence the crystals of ice formed in the fibres of the beef are sufficiently large to burst open. When thawed, such meat is wet, loses a good deal of juice as "drip" and is altered in texture.

By means of chilling it has been possible to import beef from Argentina—a journey of about three weeks. The journey from Australia—about six weeks—is too long for beef which has simply been chilled. By pumping carbon dioxide, to a concentration of 10%, into the refrigerated holds of the ships, the activity of micro-organisms is further retarded and by this "gas storage" beef can now be imported from Australia.

The method of "quick freezing" which can be used for small pieces of meat gives least loss in nutritive value.

Fish

Fish is a more delicate flesh than beef or mutton and, unless quickly frozen at a very low temperature so that very small ice crystals are formed, is liable to be spoilt in texture on thawing and cooking. By freezing fish in brine a temperature of $-11°C$ is reached. This is often done on the fishing trawlers themselves.

For the transport of fish from the big fishing ports such as Hull, Grimsby, Fleetwood and Aberdeen, fish is placed in boxes with ice and salt and carried to all parts of the country by express fish trains in vans containing solid carbon dioxide (dry ice).

Herrings have recently been "quick-frozen" by the "Birdseye method" in which they are packed ungutted into trays, placed between cold plates and there frozen solid. In this form they are packed in special cartons and placed in cold store. In another method, known as the "airblast method," the herrings are packed ungutted and then passed into a tunnel through which currents of cold air blast the fish until they are frozen and then they are stored at $-32°$ C.

In both methods there is the shortest possible time between landing the fish and processing it so that decay and bacterial growth are reduced to a minimum.

Eggs

Freezing is not a suitable method for preserving shell eggs, the shell is apt to break and the membrane surrounding the yolk to burst. Consequently imported shell eggs are chilled instead of frozen. In addition, the humidity of the air is carefully regulated to prevent mould growths. Alternatively, the eggs are stored in a high concentration of carbon dioxide which prevents mould growth and bacterial development. This latter method is known as "gas storage." Canned liquid eggs can be frozen. Such eggs are used by confectioners for baking.

Food	*Preparation*	*Length of time for keeping*
VEGETABLES	They are prepared as for cooking, are then blanched in boiling water and cooled in iced water for an equal time, before being drained and packed.	1 year
French beans	Blanch for 1 minute if sliced. Blanch for 2 minutes if cut.	
Carrots	Only small young ones should be used. They are peeled after blanching for 5 minutes.	
Cauliflower	Blanch for 3 minutes.	
Peas	,, ,, 1 minute.	
Sprouts	Only small tight buds are used. They should be blanched for 3 minutes.	
FRUIT		
Berries	(a) Pack in castor sugar using 250 g to 1 kilo fruit. Raspberries can be packed without sugar. (b) Cover fruit with cold sugar solution (500 g sugar to 1 litre water). About 150 g syrup should cover 250 g fruit. A ½ inch (1 cm) space should be left above liquid to allow for expansion and the surface should be covered with waxed paper to exclude air.	1 year
Peaches	Blanch ½ minute, cool in water. Peel, cut in half, remove stone, proceed as with (b) above.	
Plums and other stoned fruit	Remove stone, proceed as with (b) above.	
Oranges	Wrap in polythene bags and freeze whole.	

Food	*Preparation*	*Length of time for keeping*
MEAT		
Joints	Wrap thoroughly. Expel as much air as possible from around joint to prevent discoloration.	Beef 12 months Lamb 12 months Pork 9 months
Cuts	Place two thicknesses of greaseproof paper or plastic between each cut, protect any sharp bones, wrap carefully.	Sausage 6 weeks Bacon 4–6 weeks Mince 8 weeks
Offal	Clean thoroughly, freeze quickly.	8 weeks
Whole chicken and other fowl	Prepare as for roasting, wrap giblets separately. Put inside bird if it is to be kept for 3 months; freeze separately if bird is to be kept longer.	Chicken 12 months Ducks 6 months Giblets 3 months
Jointed fowl	Joint, Pack on metal or fibre tray, cover with foil and polythene.	
FISH		
Whole	Scale, gut, wash and dry. Freeze until firm, dip into icy cold salted water until coated with ice. Wrap in polythene; freeze.	White 6–12 months Oily 4 months
Joints	Wrap and then over wrap.	
BREAD		
Bakers bread	Freeze in waxed paper	1 week
Home-baked	Freeze wrapped in polythene.	6 months
CAKES		
Plain	Freeze wrapped in polythene. Decorate or fill after defrosting.	6 months
Iced	Freeze and then wrap.	6 months
PASTRY	Freeze-wrapped uncooked.	3 months
CHOUX PASTRY	Cook, wrap, then freeze. Fill after defrosting.	6 months
COOKED FOODS	Make cool and freeze as quickly as possible. Under-season slightly and do not thicken sauces as much as usual.	2 months

Milk

There is not much large scale use made of freezing or chilling as methods of preserving milk. It is possible, however, to serve fresh milk on board ship by storing it at 0° C. Milk will keep fresh for long periods in a home refrigerator. Butter and cheese can also be chilled but both must be wrapped to exclude air and prevent the growth of moulds and oxidation of the fat.

Fruits

The preservation of fruit during transport and storage is governed by the fact that the fruit is a living organism and as such is constantly changing. These changes can be slowed down by low temperatures but great care has to be taken not to cause unpleasant flavours, loss of colour and rupture of the cells which allows juice to be lost and the fruit to become soft.

Freezing in syrup prevents browning during storage provided the fruit is completely immersed. Raspberries, gooseberries and red currants can be successfully frozen in this way. Plums and cherries are liable to discolour when thawed out after being frozen in syrup.

Many fruits are chilled but certain precautions must be taken not to over-chill so as not to damage or kill the fruit. Apples, for example, must be wrapped in oiled paper to prevent the disease known as "scald." Different fruits, and even different varieties of the same fruit, must be chilled to different temperatures. Some fruits, such as tomatoes and bananas, are picked green and allowed to ripen during the journey and in warehouses on arrival.

The use of gas storage along with chilling delays the ripening of fruit still further and is being increasingly used for home-grown fruit. The concentration of carbon dioxide used is round about 5%.

In the modern "frozen pack," "frosted food," or "Birdseye method," the fruit is placed in containers and frozen quickly at −34° to −52° C, and stored between −18° C and −23° C. This quick-freezing process is particularly suitable for strawberries, raspberries, gooseberries and currants.

Vegetables

Asparagus, green peas, runner beans, sprouts and broad beans, sprouting broccoli and sweet corn have been successfully preserved by the quick-freeze method. They are first scalded to prevent enzyme actions which go on in raw vegetables even at low temperatures and then quickly frozen at −34° to −52° C and stored at −18° to −23° C.

Spinach is preserved by quick-freezing and may be sieved prior to freezing.

Potatoes can be deep frozen; potato chips are particularly popular. These are briefly fried before being cooled and then frozen.

PRESERVATION BY HEAT

Bacteria, yeasts and moulds are all destroyed by heat and so are the natural enzymes of food. A temperature of 65° C is sufficient to kill the cell forms of the micro-organisms but greater heat (126° C) is necessary to destroy their spores. By destroying micro-organisms and enzymes in food by heat and then placing it in a sealed container to prevent the access of air and other micro-organisms the food should keep indefinitely. This is the principle underlying the canning and bottling of foods.

This method of preservation was invented by a French chef, Nicolas Appert, in 1810, as a result of the offer of a prize by the French Government, for improved methods of preserving foods during the Napoleonic Wars. It is interesting to note that margarine was invented by Mège-Mouries in 1870 in a similar competition organised by the French Government during the Franco-German War.

Appert used glass bottles in which he covered the food with water and cooked it for several hours before sealing them with special waxed corks which were wired on to the bottles. Since Appert's time there have been great advances made, but his principles were sound and the improvements have been in technique and detail rather than in new principles. Canning has been developed where cans have replaced glass bottles. At first cans were hand-made and then machine-made. The first type had a hole in the lid which had to be sealed with solder. The hole allowed steam to escape during cooking which drove out the air and by sealing while hot a vacuum was produced in the tin. The open-top or "sanitary" can is sealed by machinery and no solder is needed. The lid is fixed while the food is hot by bonding the edges of the top of the can and the flange of the lid by a double seamer machine to give an airtight seal.

The sheet steel used in the manufacture of cans is coated with a layer of tin to prevent chemical action between the food and the can. The cans used for such acid-containing foods as fruits and vegetables are also lacquered or enamelled to give additional protection. The heating or processing of the foods is now done by superheated steam in a vacuum (vacuum pans) instead of in open pans such as Appert used. In this way, higher temperatures can be used to destroy micro-organisms without spoiling the appearance, flavour and food value, particularly the vitamin value, of foods. Chemical preservatives are now seldom used in canned foods. They are unnecessary.

Because of these improvements in methods of manufacture decomposition of canned foods is rare, but if a tin bulges outwards it is a sign of the production of gas inside the tin. Should a canned food show by its appearance or smell the least sign of decomposition it should be discarded.

Because of the ease of handling, cans have largely replaced bottles as a commercial method of preservation, but the housewife still uses bottles for bottling fruits. She processes the food at a lower temperature and relies on the acid of the fruit and added sugar, or added acid when pickling, to help to preserve the food. Home canning apparatus is available, but with the temperature the housewife reaches it is normally recommended that she should not try to can either meat or fish.

The nutritive effects of both bottling and canning vary with the product. With meat and fish there may be a high loss of vitamin B if sodium nitrate is added, and there will in any case be some loss as a result of the high temperature. The loss of vitamin C from fruit will depend on the acidity of the fruit, but will only be about 25–30% provided the juice is eaten too. The loss of vitamin C from vegetables is likely to be higher and may amount to 70%.

MEAT CANNING

As an example of meat canning the following processes are involved in the production of corned beef.

It is first cut up into small pieces and scalded in boiling water for fifteen minutes. The fat is skimmed off the liquid which is then concentrated in vacuum pans to produce meat extracts such as Oxo and Bovril. The scalded meat is pickled in a solution of common salt and sodium nitrate or sodium nitrite. The latter changes the unappetising colour of the boiled beef to a more attractive pink colour. The pickling solution is drained off, the meat packed into cans and then sterilised at high temperature in the cans in which it is packed.

Other forms of meat, e.g., mutton, pork and poultry, are canned in a similar way.

Fish

Fish such as salmon are cleaned, cut into suitable portions and parboiled after packing into cans. The cans are sealed, while still hot, and processed.

Sardines, which are immature fish of the pilchard family, are first fried in oil and then canned in oil or tomato sauce before processing.

Eggs

Shell eggs are not suitable for canning and processing. Canned liquid eggs are used sometimes by confectioners for baking purposes.

Milk

The preparation of evaporated or condensed milk has already been described. (See page 110.)

Fruits

The cans are packed with fresh graded fruit and filled with boiling water or sugar syrup. The lid is sealed on while still hot so that air will have been driven out by the steam. The sealed cans are then processed so as to sterilise and cook the fruit.

Vegetables

Vegetables are washed, cut up into suitable sizes, and then scalded or blanched. They are then packed into cans, covered with boiling water, sealed while still hot so as to produce a partial vacuum, and finally processed.

BOTTLING

The principles involved are, of course, similar to those of canning but the following points should be noted:

(a) *The Fruit.* Soft fruits, except gooseberries, should be of good colour, ripe and firm. Gooseberries should be bottled when green and slightly under-ripe. Most stone-fruits should be firm-ripe. The fruit should be picked while dry and bottled as fresh as possible. It is advisable to grade the fruit according to size and ripeness, for the time necessary for cooking will depend to some extent on the size and ripeness of the fruit. The fruit should be packed as tightly as possible and the bottles well filled.

(b) *The Bottles.* Before use the bottles should be perfectly cleaned in order to sterilise them thoroughly. The two commonest types of bottle in use for the preservation of fruit are clip bottles, e.g., Snap Closure, and screw band bottles, e.g., Kilner.

Clip bottles have lacquered tin lids fitted with rubber bands. During sterilisation they are held in position by metal spring clips. While the fruit is being heated the pressure inside the bottles increases sufficiently to lift the lids slightly and allow steam and air to escape. During cooling, the spring clip holds the lids firmly in position while the steam inside the bottles condenses to water and so creates a partial vacuum.

Screw band bottles have lacquered tin bands to hold the glass lids in position on the rubber bands placed round the rims of the bottles. During the heating the screw bands are fitted loosely so as to allow the escape of steam and air. During cooling the bands are screwed down tightly so as to hold the lids in position until a vacuum is formed when the steam condenses.

(c) *The Sterilisation.* Having been packed properly into suitable bottles the fruit should now be covered with either water or sugar syrup. Of the two, sugar syrup is preferable as the sugar impregnates the fruit during sterilisation and storing, and helps to preserve the fresh fruit flavour. The most suitable strength of sugar syrup is one containing 400–650 g per litre of water.

The rubber rings, lids and clips or screw bands are now placed in position and the fruit sterilised. Various methods can be used. The bottles can be placed on a false bottom of wood or cloth in a deep pan, zinc bath or bucket and completely covered with water. The water is heated slowly to simmering point in about 1¼ hours and retained at this temperature for 15 minutes. Alternatively, the bottles can be heated on an asbestos mat, sheet of cardboard or wood in a very moderate oven (about 115° C) for ¾ hour to 1 hour. In this oven method the water or sugar syrup can be added either before the heating or as boiling water or boiling sugar syrup after the heating.

Another method involves the use of the "high-dome" pressure cooker.

(d) *Testing the Seal.* After twenty-four hours remove the spring clip or screw band and lift the bottle by its lid. If the lid comes off the seal is imperfect and the fruit should be resterilised or eaten within a few days. If properly sealed, the difference between the atmospheric pressure outside the bottle and the small pressure of the partial vacuum inside the bottle will be great enough to hold the lid in position.

The home bottling of vegetables is not very common because it is a lengthy process requiring high temperatures and the use of a pressure cooker for sterilisation.

PRESERVATION BY SUGAR, SALT, ACIDS AND OTHER CHEMICAL SUBSTANCES

Micro-organisms are killed and the action of enzymes prevented by the use of high concentrations of sugar, salt and acids such as vinegar. Certain chemical substances such as boric acid, borax, sodium benzoate, sodium salicylate and formalin are poisonous to micro-organisms in even minute quantities. They were largely used as food preservatives until their random use was made illegal by the Public Health Authorities in 1925 because of their harmful effect upon the health of people eating foods preserved in this way. The preservatives of this type permitted by the Regulations are very limited and even these can only be used in restricted amounts and in certain foods such as sausages, meat pastes and dehydrated vegetables. The presence of these preservatives and the amount must be stated on the label.

However, a large range of substances are added to foods to help to preserve them: for instance sodium diacetate, sodium and calcium propionates, acetic acid, lactic acid and monocalcium phosphate are added to baked products to inhibit the growth of moulds and bacteria. Sorbic acid can be added to cheese, syrups and pie fillings to prevent the growth of moulds. Benzoic acid and sodium benzoate are commonly added to a variety of foods including margarine, fruit juices and pickles, and sulphur dioxide can be used to help to preserve dried fruits.

If one includes in this list substances that are added to prevent the oxidation of foods which may lead to unpleasant flavours, loss of colour and browning, then one must add citric, ascorbic and phosphoric acids, sodium sulphite and various complex organic substances. The presence of these preservatives, and in some cases the amount, must be stated on the label, and there is a constant check on their use and research into their possible toxicity to both humans and animals.

Meat

In the past the salting of meat was the usual method of preserving it. The meat was either rubbed with dry salt or pickled in salt solution (brine). At the present time pork is the only form of meat extensively salted. The rolled or unrolled sides of the pig, after removal of the ribs, form bacon, while the back legs form hams. The old-fashioned method still used in farmhouses is the dry-salting one in which dry salt is rubbed into the pork. The bacon or ham is afterwards hung, with or without smoking. Modern mild-cured bacon and ham are cured in brine and do not keep anything like as long as dry-salted bacon and ham. In addition to common salt, a little sodium nitrite or potassium nitrate (saltpetre) is used. It acts as a preservative and gives the bacon or ham an attractive red colour.

Micro-organisms cannot grow in the high concentrations of salt in bacon and ham and, in addition, the salt absorbs water from the meat and so partly dries it. The keeping qualities are enhanced by smoking with sawdusts of hard woods such as oak and beech. The meat absorbs substances from the smoke which have an antiseptic action. It is also altered in flavour and dried further.

Fish

Salt is very frequently used to preserve fish. Cod is salted in large quantities in Newfoundland, Iceland and Greenland. In Great Britain fish is both salted and smoked. The kipper is herring which has been split and salted before smoking. Bloaters are similar to kippers but have more salt added. Red herrings have a further addition of salt and are smoked for ten days. Haddocks were first cured at Findon, a small fishing village near Aberdeen, from which the name Finnon Haddock is derived. Salmon which has been salted and smoked is eaten without further cooking.

Eggs

We have already seen that liquid eggs are canned and used for confectionery purposes.

Chemical preservatives used for shell eggs act in a different way. Micro-organisms can be prevented from attacking the food materials in the egg by blocking up the pores in the shell. This can be done by "pickling" them in solutions of water-glass (sodium silicate), lime or borax. Alternatively, the eggs can be sealed by coating them with melted paraffin wax or special varnishes such as Oteg.

Pickling is the most suitable domestic method of preserving eggs. The eggs can be pickled when they are plentiful and used when they are scarce. A "pickled" egg will remain fit for use for twelve months. When a pickled egg is boiled the shell almost invariably cracks because the pores of the shell are sealed and the expansion of the air-chamber during heating causes a sufficient internal pressure to break the shell. This can be prevented by making a small hole through the broad end of the egg into the air-chamber by means of a pin or needle.

Milk

The use of chemical preservatives of any type in liquid milk or cream is prohibited by Public Health Regulations. Condensed milk is sweetened and its keeping qualities enhanced by the addition of sugar.

The salt added to butter, margarine and cheese not merely gives flavour but acts as a preservative as well. Although very little salt is used, the amount of water, margarine and cheese is so small that a concentrated salt solution is produced. It should be realised that, in a sense, butter and cheese are preserved forms of milk. Both keep much better than the milk from which they are prepared.

Vegetables

Kidney beans and runner beans can be preserved by storing them between layers of salt, but the usual chemical preservative for vegetables is vinegar. The sharp sour taste of vinegar is due to the presence of acetic acid and it is this acid which prevents the activities of micro-organisms in pickled vegetables.

The vinegar is first boiled with spices and salt and after cooling is poured over the onions or walnuts. Piccalilli contains cauliflower and other vegetables. Mustard and ginger are used as well as vinegar, salt and spices. Chutneys of fruits and vegetables are made with sugar, vinegar and salt as preservatives, and ginger and spices as flavourings.

Fruit

Very large amounts of fruit are preserved by means of sugar in the form of jams, jellies, marmalades, candied peels, and glacé or crystallised fruits. By producing a high concentration of sugar in and around the fruit the growth of moulds and yeasts is prevented.

Jam

Fresh fruit contains fibre, water, sugars, fruit-acids and a gum-like substance known as pectin. This pectin is of great importance in jam-making because it is to pectin that the setting of jam is due. Successful "gel" formation depends upon the extraction of as much pectin as possible and fruit acids are necessary to do this.

Fruits such as plums, damsons, currants and gooseberries are easily made into jam because they contain large proportions of both pectin and fruit acids. On the other hand, strawberries, pears, rhubarb and marrow contain very little pectin or acid and are consequently difficult to make into jam. Acid substances such as lemon juice, tartaric acid, cream of tartar, citric acid, gooseberry juice or red currant juice are frequently added to such fruits. The presence of acid in the fruit improves the colour and flavour of the jam and also prevents "graining" or crystallisation of the sugar in the jam when it is stored. This graining is prevented by the "inversion" of some of the cane sugar to invert sugar (glucose and fructose) during the boiling of the jam. Strawberries, cherries and rhubarb can be made to form excellent jam by the addition of pectin from other fruits. This can be done by making the jam of two fruits, e.g., strawberry and apple, or by adding home-made pectin or commercial pectin preparations.

Home-made pectin stock can be prepared from such pectin-rich fruits as apples, red currants or gooseberries, by simmering 1½ kg of fruit with a ½ litre of water until tender. The fruit is then mashed and strained through a scalded jelly bag and left to drain. After draining, the pulp in the jelly bag is again simmered for about an hour and finally strained. The two extracts thus obtained are then mixed. The mixture can be tested for pectin by pouring a sample into methylated spirits. Pectin is insoluble in alcohol and is precipitated as a jelly-like clot. If only a poor clot is obtained the extract should be further concentrated. Finally the extract is bottled and stored for use with fruit poor in pectin.

There are a number of commercial pectin preparations such as Certo, Zett and Pexicon. When these are used for jam-making the time of boiling is very much reduced, the yield of jam is greater, the fresh fruit colour and flavour are more readily preserved and a well set jam is ensured. Such concentrated pectin preparations should, however, be used with care and the enclosed directions accurately followed. Otherwise the jam will be too stiff or the delicate fruit flavour ruined.

The fruit used for jam-making should be perfectly fresh and firm ripe. It is at this stage that fruits are richest in pectin and acid. Over-ripe fruits contain a diminishing amount of pectin and acid and are liable to mould growth and loss of colour and flavour.

After cleaning, the fruit should be cooked for some time before the sugar is added. The length of time for this cooking varies according to the fruit used: from 10–15 minutes with such fruits as raspberries, to 30–45 minutes, with addition of water, in the case of plums, damsons and blackcurrants. It is during this preliminary cooking that the pectin is extracted and in the case of fruits deficient in fruit acids it is at this stage that additional acid should be added.

The fruit is sufficiently cooked when a good pectin clot is obtained with the following test. A teaspoonful of jam free from seeds and skins is placed in a tumbler or cup and three teaspoonfuls of methylated spirits added to it. The mixture is shaken gently and left for a minute. If the fruit contains sufficient pectin a transparent jelly-like clot of pectin will be formed and, when poured into another tumbler or cup, will remain in one piece. A poor clot may divide into two or three lumps and a very poor clot into numerous small pieces.

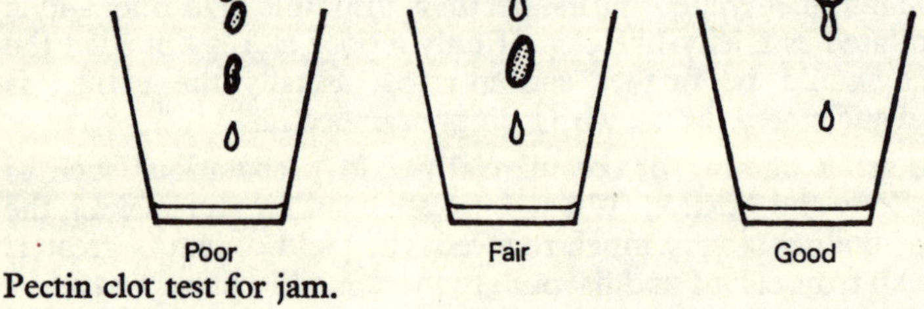

Pectin clot test for jam.

When a good pectin clot has been obtained by this test, the fruit is ready for the addition of sugar. The most suitable type is a good quality granulated sugar. As a general rule a kilogramme of sugar should be added for each kilogramme of fruit. The mixture should be stirred until all the sugar has dissolved and then boiled as rapidly as possible without stirring as air bubbles and scum may get mixed up with the jam and spoil its appearance.

This boiling period will vary from about three to twenty minutes according to the kind and quantity of fruit and the shape and size of the pan. The object is to reduce this period of boiling with sugar to a minimum in order to produce a jam with a fresh fruit flavour, good colour and firm set. Boiling too long will weaken the setting qualities of the pectin and some of the sugar may be caramelised and so spoil the flavour and colour of the finished jam. On the other hand, if the jam is not boiled long enough an insufficient amount of sugar will be inverted to prevent the jam going sugary on keeping.

The following tests may be made, to find when the jam has reached setting point:

(1) *Cold Plate Test*
A sample of the jam is poured from a wooden spoon on to a cold plate. When the jam has reached setting point the surface of the sample should set quickly and crinkle when pushed with the finger.

(2) *Flake Test*
A sample of the jam is taken out on a wooden spoon and turned horizontally until the sample is partly cooled. The jam is then allowed to drop from the edge of the spoon. If the drops run together into flakes which break off cleanly, setting point is reached.

(3) *Temperature Test*
Provided a sugar-boiler's thermometer is available, this is the most reliable test. When the jam boils at 105°C it will set on cooling.

(4) *Weight Test*
This test consists in weighing the pan and its contents (without spoon) on a suitable spring balance until the weight of added sugar forms 60% of the weight of the jam. Thus, if the recipe contains 3 kg of sugar, setting point is reached when the weight of jam

reaches $\frac{3}{1} \times \frac{100}{60} = 5$ kg. It must be remembered, of course, that the weight of the jam does not include the weight of the pan.

When setting point is reached, the jam should be removed from the source of heat and any scum quickly skimmed off. The jam should then be quickly poured into clean, dry, warm jars which should be filled quite up to the top to allow for considerable shrinkage on cooling. Wax discs, waxed side downwards, should be placed on the surface of the jam to prevent it absorbing moisture from the air and so giving moulds and yeasts a chance to grow. Finally, the jars should be tied down with jam covers to prevent the access of moulds and yeasts and stored in a cool, dry, airy place.

A really good jam should be well set but not too stiff. It should be clear and bright in colour and have a distinct fruity flavour. It should be capable of storage without fermenting or going either mouldy or sugary. Finally, the fruit should be soft of flesh and tender of skin and should be evenly distributed throughout the jars.

The following are the chief faults found in jams.

(a) Mould on Jam

Jam may go mouldy because of any of the following:

(1) Too little sugar has been used.
(2) Storage in a damp warm place.
(3) The use of wet or inferior fruit.
(4) A wet summer which predisposes fruit to mould growth.
(5) Incomplete destruction of mould spores during boiling.

(b) Fermentation of Jam

This is caused by yeasts converting some of the sugar into alcohol. Jams may ferment because:

(1) Too little sugar has been used.
(2) Underboiling has resulted in too large a yield of jam. If 3 kg of sugar are used the yield of jam should not be more than 5 kg.

(c) Graining of Jam

Some of the sugar may crystallise out and the jam go sugary because:

(1) Too much sugar has been used.
(2) Too little of the sugar has been inverted. This may be because

the jam was not boiled long enough to allow the acids of the fruit to invert sufficient of the sugar or the fruit may have contained too little acid to bring about sufficient inversion.

(*d*) *Other Faults*

(1) The fruit may have risen to the top of the jar. This is particularly common with strawberry jam and marmalade. It can be avoided by allowing the fruit to cool slightly until it begins to stiffen and then stirring it gently before pouring it into jars.

(2) The jam may be dull and cloudy in appearance and lacking in fresh fruit flavour. This may be due to stirring during the boiling with sugar or to over boiling and caramelisation of some of the sugar, or because the scum of coagulated proteins from the fruit has not been removed.

Fruit Jellies

The preparation of fruit jellies depends upon the same principles as those of jam. With the exception of strawberries, cherries and pears, which are deficient in pectin and acid, all the common fruits can be made into jellies. The most suitable are currants, gooseberries, loganberries and quinces and such wild fruits as elderberries, bilberries, blackberries, sloes and crab apples. The wild berries set better if mixed with cooking apples.

The fresh firm-ripe fruit is first washed but it is unneccessary to remove stalks, leaves, etc., as they will be removed during straining. Large fruits, such as apples and plums, should be cut into small pieces. The fruit is then cooked in water, the amount of water depending upon the type of fruit. The cooking should be slow and the fruit simmered until tender when the maximum amount of pectin and acid will be extracted. The test for pectin is the same as with jam and when a good clot is obtained the pulp is strained through a scalded jelly bag.

The juice is now heated and skimmed and sugar added at the rate 200 g to $\frac{1}{4}$ litre of juice. The juice is stirred until all the sugar is dissolved and then boiled as rapidly as possible without stirring. The jelly will set, as in the case of jam, when the added sugar content has reached 60%. The same test for setting point can be used as with jam (except the weight test). When setting point is reached the hot jelly is immediately poured into clean, dry, warm jars until completely filled. Wax circles are placed on the surface of the jelly while still hot and the jars tied down after cooling. The jars should then be stored in a cool, dry, airy place.

This type of fruit jelly should not be confused with the commercial type made of gelatine, coloured and flavoured to resemble some particular fruit.

Marmalade

The preparation of marmalade from such citrus fruits as oranges, lemons, grapefruits and limes is so similar in method and principles to jams and jellies that the following details only need be mentioned.

The thick rinds of citrus fruits require boiling for at least two hours and the addition of water is essential during the cooking. It is important that the white inner skin or "pith" and pips should be cooked along with the rest of the fruit since most of the pectin is in them and not in the juice. If considered desirable, the pith and pips can be placed in a muslin bag and cooked along with the marmalade and then taken out before the sugar is added. In this way the valuable pectin is extracted without spoiling the appearance of the marmalade by the presence of white pith in it.

Composition of Jams

The composition of jam varies but the following table gives a general average composition.

Water	28%
Sucrose	36%
Invert Sugar	33%
Fruit Acids	0·75%
Pectin	0·5–0·75%
Seeds and Fibres (exclusive of stones)	1–2%

Under the Fruit Standards (Preserves) Order, 1953, commercial jams must have a minimum fruit content and a minimum soluble solids content, i.e., added sugar together with the small amount of sugar from the fruit. The legal minimum fruit content of the finished jam varies with the particular fruit e.g., 25% for blackcurrant, 30% for raspberry and 38% for strawberry. The minimum legal percentage of soluble solids is 68·5 (65 if the jam is sealed in containers while the contents are hot with a closure capable of maintaining a partial vacuum on cooling i.e., hermetically sealed). These prescribed minimum standards ensure jams of good quality, and jams are not now adulterated with vegetables and cheap varieties of fruit as sometimes happened in the past. Jam must not now contain any fruit other than that named on the label. It must consist only of the named fruits, sugar, pectin and water.

Candied Peels, Glacé and Crystallised Fruits and Flowers

The chief candied peels are those of the lemon, orange, citron, grapefruit and lime. The fruits are cut in two and the pulp removed. The "caps" are soaked in brine to soften them and then washed in water to remove the salt. They are placed in tanks of weak sugar syrup and absorb some of the sugar. By passing into stronger and stronger sugar syrups the caps become saturated with sugar. Finally, they are drained, dried and candied by heating for several hours. The heating sets the sugar and hardens the caps.

Glacé or crystallised fruits, such as cherries, first of all have their stones removed and then they are cooked in weak sugar syrup until soft and finally rolled in melted sugar.

Crystallised ginger is made from the underground stem (rhizome) of the ginger plant by first cleaning and then cooking it in weak sugar syrup. The much more common ground ginger is made by grinding the dried rhizome.

Angelica and Sweet Parma violets and rose petals are crystallised in a similar way and used for decorative purposes in confectionery.

CORRECT STORAGE

In concluding this important chapter we would point out that, although not regarded as preservation in the strict sense of the term, the keeping of food fresh as long as possible by proper storage in the home is really a form of temporary preservation. Full use should be made of refrigerators whenever available for such foods as milk, meat, fish, eggs, butter, margarine and fats. Other simple methods of keeping milk fresh have already been given. Similar methods can be used for butter, margarine and fats.

Cheese should be kept cool and dry.

Bread should be kept wrapped in a clean cloth on an airy shelf or in a clean, dry, ventilated bin. New bread should be quite cold before being put away.

Green vegetables should be kept away from the air in an airtight container, e.g., a large saucepan with the lid on.

Root vegetables should be kept cool and moist. Potatoes should be kept in a dry, cool, well-ventilated place and not exposed to a bright light which may make them turn green and taste bitter when cooked. If conditions are too warm, potatoes may blacken on cooking. Potatoes should not be stored near anything with a strong smell as they can absorb other flavours and should be handled with more care than they often receive as they bruise fairly easily and consequently turn black when cooked.

Cereals, pulses and flour should be kept perfectly dry, preferably in glass, plastic or metal containers with lids.

16 The Cooking of Foods

THE REASONS FOR COOKING FOOD

The practice of cooking meat and other foods has grown up with civilisation and the general advance in refinement of taste. Primitive man depended upon uncooked raw food. Civilised man is the only living creature that does not eat his food raw.

The purposes of cooking food can be summarised as follows:

(1) To improve its appearance.
(2) To develop new flavours and so stimulate appetite and the flow of digestive juices.
(3) To make the food more digestible.
(4) To destroy micro-organisms and parasites and so make the food keep longer.

The following methods of cooking are usually distinguished: stewing, boiling, braising, baking, roasting, grilling, frying and steaming. All of them, of course, involve the use of heat which may be applied to the food in three different ways.

(1) Dry heat applied directly to the food in roasting, baking, grilling and braising.
(2) Moist heat applied by means of hot water or steam in stewing, boiling and steaming.
(3) High temperatures applied by means of hot fat in frying.

Before dealing separately with each method of cooking we must first discuss the action of heat upon the nutrients of food, carbohydrates, fats, proteins, minerals and vitamins.

The Effects of Cooking on the Main Nutrients

Carbohydrates

Cooking is essential if starch is to be digested. Uncooked starch in flour, potatoes, rice, oatmeal and so on is in the form of "cells" or granules with an outer layer which our digestive juices cannot easily penetrate. With moist heat the starch cells swell up and burst and the starch is said to be gelatinised. In this form it can easily be converted by our digestive juices into glucose and completely absorbed. Gelatinisation of starch takes place when bread is baked, potatoes boiled, custard powder made into custards with boiling milk and so on. With dry heat starch is converted into dextrin which is easily digested.

Cane sugar in acid solutions as in stewed fruits and jams is inverted into invert sugar (glucose and fructose). The formation of caramel by the action of heat on sugar alters the flavour and colour of many foods during cooking.

Fats

Unless fats are heated to very high temperatures the only changes which take place are that they melt to oils and lose any moisture they contain. Butter may lose some of its more volatile fats and thus lose its superior flavour and become harder and more tallowy. At very high temperatures, such as in frying, some of the fat may be decomposed into fatty acids and glycerin, and even some of the glycerin decomposed into acrolein, which has an irritating effect on the digestive organs.

Proteins

Proteins are "set" or coagulated by heat. This is most easily seen in the white of a boiled egg. In addition, proteins shrink on heating. This is seen in the shrinkage of meat during roasting owing to the contraction of the protein of the muscle fibres. Lightly coagulated protein is more digestible than raw protein, e.g., a lightly boiled egg is more digestible than a raw egg, but over-coagulation makes protein less digestible and reduces its food value.

Minerals

Dry heat has little effect upon the minerals of food. Boiling may result in the loss of some of the soluble magnesium, potassium and sodium salts but this is of little consequence because we get plenty of these minerals in our diet. The more valuable calcium and iron are practically unaffected by boiling. In fact, their amounts in foods are sometimes increased by the absorption of calcium from hard water and iron from the utensils.

Vitamins

Vitamins A and D are insoluble in water and can withstand the temperatures of ordinary methods of cooking so that cooked foods contain as much of these vitamins as the raw foods.

Some of the vitamin B_1 (thiamine) may be lost in cooking water since it is very soluble. It is destroyed at very high temperatures particularly in the presence of bicarbonate of soda. Riboflavin and nicotinic acid are not much affected by ordinary methods of cooking in spite of the fact that they are soluble in water and destroyed at high temperatures. Pressure cooking and the corning of beef are likely to cause some loss of both these vitamins.

Vitamin C (ascorbic acid) is the vitamin most easily dissolved out of foods and destroyed by heat. As previously pointed out (page 58), this loss is greatest if the heating is prolonged, or takes place in the presence of air, or if the vegetables are grated, or the boiling started from the cold. By careful cooking the loss of ascorbic acid in vegetables can be reduced to a minimum.

METHODS OF COOKING

Roasting or Baking is the cooking of food in a closed oven. Most of the heat reaches the outside of the food by radiation, but where it is in contact with the tin it will be by conduction. The heat reaches the inside of the food by conduction and only penetrates slowly, so that when roasting or baking it is important to see that the outside is not overcooked whilst allowing the necessary time for heat to penetrate inside.

The heat in an oven can be varied from about 200°C to about 500°C, and is of course a dry heat. If a damp heat is required, the food can be enclosed in foil, but the cooking effects resemble steaming when this is done.

The considerable heat involved seals the outside of the food, will partially denature the surface protein of meat and fish, will destroy some of the thiamine in foods, and will convert some surface starch to dextrins.

Grilling is really very quick small-scale roasting, and involves the use of a very hot radiating surface which only cooks the food on the top. It is only suitable for thin samples of food, or for cooking the surface of a dish.

Stewing. In stewing, the food is placed in water and the temperature of the water is raised until it just begins to bubble at the side of the pan—about 96° C. The food is cooked very slowly and any nutrients that are soluble are extracted and go into the water. Vitamin C will be destroyed by the prolonged cooking.

Boiling. In boiling the food is placed in water which is kept on boiling point. Any nutrients that are soluble are extracted and go into the water, but as it is a faster method of cooking than stewing, there is less destruction of vitamin C.

Steaming. Steaming is cooking in the steam from boiling water in a steamer, which has a tight-fitting lid to prevent loss of steam. The temperature is the same as that of boiling water (100° C) and the results similar to boiling except that there is less loss of minerals and extractives though more than in roasting, grilling or frying.

Pressure Cooking. Pressure cooking involves the use of steam under pressure. In most pressure cookers the pressure can be varied so that the temperature used will vary from 100° C to 138° C. By using a higher temperature for cooking, the time needed for cooking can be much reduced. There is little difference in the effects on the nutrients between normal steaming and pressure cooking as the higher temperature and shorter time more or less balance each other, though if anything there is likely to be slightly less loss of thiamine and vitamin C in pressure cooking.

Despite the variations in size and design of the pressure cookers, the cooking principles are the same in all cases. They are based on the fact that the lid is completely sealed or locked on the pan so that no steam can escape until the desired steam pressure is reached. With increase in pressure there is a proportionate increase in temperature.

Under these conditions the food cooks more quickly than by other methods. The saving in cooking time is, in fact, considerable. It naturally varies with different foods but is obviously greatest with those foods which normally require long slow cooking. On the average, cooking times are reduced by about two-thirds and occasionally by three-quarters or even more. Detailed instructions are issued with each cooker and all cooking times must be strictly followed or the food will quickly be overcooked. The time taken for cooking is always reckoned after cooking pressure is reached. The time taken to expel air and build up the steam pressure varies according to whether the pressure cooker is heated on a gas, electric, oil or heat-storage cooker, or on a kitchen range. An average time is 6–8 minutes. Once the cooking pressure is reached, the heat can be reduced to simmering point for the rest of the cooking time so that as well as economy in time there is considerable economy of fuel.

It is unnecessary to go into details here about the use of pressure cookers since these differ very slightly with different makes. The manufacturers' directions for each cooker should be closely followed. These general points which apply to all types of pressure saucepans should be noted:

1. It is essential to put ½ to 1 cup of water in the cooker to form steam.

2. The small rack or false base provided should be used for all cooking except soups and stews.

3. Although the pressure saucepans are strong and durable and can withstand much higher pressures than the normal pressures used, the pressure control device needs careful attention. If this device becomes clogged up so that steam cannot escape, the cooker may become overheated and the safety plug may be blown out. Thus, the cleaning of the cooker after use is an important routine proceeding.

4. As soon as the cooking time has expired the cooker should be taken off the heat, and with the exception of a few foods such as soups, stews or meat, cooled under the cold water tap for a few seconds. This immediately reduces the pressure and prevents over cooking of the food. When this has been done, the pressure control lever or other device should be lifted and the pressure released. In some cookers it is impossible to take off the lid until the pressure has been completely reduced while with others it is not comfortable or safe to do so because of the escaping steam.

5. The cooker should not be filled too full or surplus steam may not be able to escape through the pressure control device. Two-thirds full is sufficient for solids and only half-full for liquids.

6. Food should not be left on the rubber band which helps to make the seal. The rubber band may be damaged and so cause a leak.

7. The small-type pressure cookers are not suitable for preserving vegetables, meat or fish because of their smallness and because the pressure claimed by the manufacturers is only approximate.

It seems obvious that the natural flavours of all foods will be more completely retained by pressure cookery than by any other method of cooking. No aroma can escape during cooking, and salt and seasonings should be added in only very small quantities.

It is also clear that, provided it is not overcooked, the colour of meat is retained and bones used for stock are softened and presumably make the stock richer in calcium. Mineral salts will probably be leached out less than in ordinary methods of cooking, because of the small amount of water used and the short time of cooking. Vitamins A and D will not be affected by pressure cooking. Vitamin B_1 and vitamin C are the two nutrients most likely to be affected. Recent experiments suggest that the detrimental effect of the high temperature of pressure cooking is more than counterbalanced by the very short time of cooking with very little water and in the absence of air. It seems safe to say that pressure cooking of vegetables is unlikely to lead to greater destruction of vitamin C than ordinary methods of cooking and that there is less loss of vitamin B.

It is interesting to note that the pressure cooker provides the only means of cooking at high altitudes.

Braising. Braising is a combination of steaming and roasting, and is used mainly as a method of cooking meat. There is a loss of some of the soluble nutrients into the water, but as this is used for gravy the actual loss is only of some of the vitamin B_1 (thiamine) that is destroyed by the heat.

High Frequency or Microwave Cooking. Uses high frequency electric waves which agitate the molecules and cause the food to heat up. The food cooks rapidly from within outwards, but the waves can only penetrate to a depth of about two inches. If a brown appearance is wanted, food must be "finished" under the grill or in a conventional oven.

Frying. We have already seen (page 80) that the smoking temperatures to which fats are heated for frying are much higher than the temperature of boiling water; 182–204°C compared with 100°C. At these higher temperatures there is very rapid evaporation of water, and shrinkage and coagulation of the proteins. Practically all the minerals and extractives are left behind. There is less loss than with roasting or grilling and much less than with boiling or stewing. Fried foods are thus well flavoured.

The proteins are coagulated so rapidly that only small pieces of food should be fried. With large pieces there is a danger that the outer layers may be over-coagulated while the interior is still uncooked. To prevent over-coagulation of the outside proteins and the absorption of too much fat, many foods are coated with batter, egg and bread crumbs or flour and milk, before frying.

It is usual to distinguish two types of frying—shallow or dry frying, and deep fat frying. In shallow frying the food is cooked in a frying pan with very little fat. It is really baking rather than frying, the amount of fat used merely preventing the food sticking to the pan. Shallow frying is suitable for foods which already contain a good deal of fat, e.g., ham, bacon and sausage.

In deep fat frying, a deep heavy pan is necessary which should contain sufficient fat to cover the food completely. A frying basket or perforated ladle is required to lower the food gently into the heated fat and to lift it out all together. Too much food should not be put into the fat at a time as this reduces the temperature of the fat and the food will not cook properly. After frying, the food should be placed on clean kitchen paper to absorb some of the grease and so keep the food crisp. Fried foods should be served quickly and eaten hot.

COOKING AND OUR MAIN FOODS

1. Meat

The objects of cooking meat are to remove its raw appearance without over-coagulating the proteins or removing the minerals and extractives, and to make the connective tissue less tough.

Roasting or baking is suitable for fairly large joints of meat which must, however, be tender, otherwise the meat is likely to become tough and dry. Besides beef, mutton and pork, poultry, game and rabbits can be roasted or baked.

The meat for roasting should be trimmed and, when necessary, boned, tied and skewered into a suitable shape. It is then put into a tin with a little dripping and placed in a very hot oven (260° C).

The meat quickly turns a brown colour owing to the destruction of the red colouring matter, haemoglobin. The proteins of the muscle fibres and the connective tissues shrink and juice is squeezed out on to the surface of the meat. A small amount of the juice falls to the bottom of the tin as drip but much more evaporates as steam and leaves the minerals and extractives on the surface. In this way the outside layers of roasted meat get their additional flavour. The evaporation of water from the meat is the chief cause of the very marked loss in weight which occurs in roasting.

As the meat becomes hotter the proteins on the outside coagulate and slow down the loss of juice from inside the joint. After this sealing process the heat should be reduced or the meat moved to a cooler part of the oven (175° C), otherwise the proteins will be over-coagulated on the outside of the joint before the heat has penetrated to the interior because meat is a very bad conductor of heat. The dripping will melt as well as some of the fat of the meat, and these, together with the drip from the meat, form the gravy. Sometimes, during the roasting, the meat is basted with the hot fat in order to prevent the outside of the joint becoming dry and hard and also to assist in the cooking. The meat may be turned over in order to cook it evenly, but, if this is done, the fork should be stuck into the fat rather than the lean part of the joint so as not to allow juice to escape.

If an open tin is used, the draught in a gas oven causes a greater loss in weight by evaporation and consequent drying of the meat than in an electric, coke or coal oven. There is less evaporation and drying in any type of oven if a closed tin is used. Consequently there is more drip and more of the minerals and extractives pass into the gravy. Thus, roasting in a closed tin gives juicier meat and richer gravy while an open tin gives a drier, better flavoured joint but poorer gravy.

Grilling is only suitable for small pieces of meat, e.g., chops, which should be tender and of the best quality. The meat is placed on a gridiron, heated very strongly and frequently turned as the proteins coagulate. The juice squeezed out during shrinkage evaporates very quickly in the great heat and leaves the minerals and extractives on the surface so that grilled meat has an excellent flavour.

The grillers on gas and electric ovens can be used for bacon, ham and sausages as well as for browning the surfaces of puddings and savouries.

Braising. Braising is a combination of steaming and roasting and is done in a closely covered vessel in the oven or on top of the stove. The stewing softens the meat and makes it more tender, while the roasting improves the flavour by browning and crisping the surface. It is thus a suitable method of cooking for tough, stringy joints of inferior flavour.

Stewing. In stewing, the meat is cut up into small pieces, placed in a small amount of water or stock in a closely covered pan to avoid loss of steam, and the liquid gently heated so as not to reach a temperature of more than 84° C. Much so-called stewing is really simmering or slow-boiling at 100° C. At the lower temperature the cooking takes place more slowly and there is little danger of over-coagulation of the proteins. A good deal of the minerals and extractives are dissolved out from the small pieces of meat. This makes them rather tasteless but this does not matter very much because the richly flavoured cooking liquid is served along with the meat. The prolonged action of heat and moisture converts much of the collagen of the connective tissues of the meat into gelatine so that the muscle fibres easily fall apart and the meat becomes tender. Stewing is thus a suitable method of cooking the cheaper, tougher cuts of meat unsuitable for roasting. Although stewing is usually started from the cold, it has been found to make no difference to the final result whether the meat is placed in cold water or hot water.

Stewing is an economical method of cooking, not only because it can be used for the cheaper cuts of meat, but also because there is no waste, as well as a saving of fuel and cooking space since potatoes and other vegetables can be cooked along with the meat as is done in Irish stew and Lancashire hot pot.

Boiling. In boiling, the meat is placed in one piece in water or stock and kept at boiling point (100° C) until cooked. It is suitable for large pieces of meat which require thorough cooking but which are not tender enough for roasting. There is the same destruction of haemoglobin and consequent change in colour as in other methods of cooking. At 60° C some of the juice is squeezed out owing to the shrinkage of the proteins of the muscle fibres and the minerals and extractives pass into the cooking water which should be used for soup or stock. The heat penetrates slowly into the interior of the meat and the proteins are coagulated. There is less danger of over-coagulation of the outside layers than in roasting and grilling but the meat is not so well-flavoured. It makes no difference to the amount of minerals and extractives lost, or to the amount of shrinkage, whether the meat is started in cold or boiling water or whether the water is just boiling or boiling vigorously.

Steaming is cooking in the steam from boiling water in a steamer which fits tightly on to a saucepan and has a tight-fitting lid to prevent loss of steam. The temperature is the same as that of boiling water (100° C) and the results similar to boiling except that there is less loss of minerals and extractives though more than in roasting, grilling or frying.

2. Fish

Fish is more easily cooked than meat. There is no need to adopt a particular method of cooking suitable for a particular cut as there is with meat. The flesh of fish is of much more even quality than meat and since it is usually cooked in small pieces the difficulties caused by the poor heat conductivity of large pieces of meat do not arise.

The changes that take place during the cooking of fish are similar to those of meat except that there is not the same marked change in colour. There is a similar evaporation of water and shrinkage and coagulation of protein causing the flesh to become firm. But the connective tissue only has collagen fibres, which are converted to gelatine on cooking and so the muscle fibres fall apart on cooking. In the case of fat fish, such as herrings, some of the fat slowly oozes away. There are less minerals and extractives in fish than in meat. Consequently, boiling and steaming, while making fish easily digestible and suitable for invalids, are apt to make it insipid in taste because of the loss of these flavouring agents. Baked, grilled or fried fish are more tasty because of the smaller losses of minerals and extractives.

Small fat fish—herrings, kippers and smoked haddock—may be grilled or shallow fried; fillets of larger fish may be deep fried; small pieces of large white fish boiled, steamed or fried. Sometimes large fish, such as salmon, are cooked whole.

3. Eggs

Eggs differ from meat and fish in that there is much less evaporation and no shrinkage on cooking. The proteins coagulate at 72°C which is much below the boiling point of water (100° C) so that it is not necessary to have boiling water to "boil" an egg. If heated above 72° C for any length of time the proteins are apt to become tough, hard and indigestible. Whether boiled, poached, or scrambled, eggs should be only lightly cooked. The high temperature of the hot fat used in frying eggs is apt to over-coagulate the proteins—we do not coat eggs with a protective batter as we do fish. Fried eggs are not suitable for invalids and young children.

4. Fruits

Sweet fruits are best eaten uncooked but green gooseberries, black currants, red currants, damsons, cooking apples and cooking pears are improved if stewed with sugar. The skins are made tender and the fruit softened. Some of the soluble ingredients and vitamins of the fruit pass into the cooking water and some of the sugar is absorbed by the fruit but since we consume the cooking water as well as the fruit this is no detriment, and because of the acids in the fruit the losses of vitamin B_1 and vitamin C are less than would otherwise be the case.

It is important to remember that not all fruit contains vitamin C and the nutritional contribution of cooked apples, plums and pears to the diet is little more than some carbohydrate and roughage.

5. Vegetables

The chief reasons for cooking vegetables are to soften the cellulose framework and to gelatinise the starch grains. The proteins of vegetables are coagulated in exactly the same way as those of animal foods. Unlike meat and fish, vegetables usually become bulkier after cooking. There is a danger that the cooking of vegetables may result in a loss of some of their mineral salts but, fortunately, the important ones, calcium and iron, are the least affected. Carotene is not likely to be lost by cooking since it is fairly stable to heat and is not soluble in water. Vitamin B_1 is not much affected by the temperatures of cooking but is very soluble in water so that much of it is likely to be lost in the cooking water. The use of bicarbonate of soda to preserve the green colour of vegetables causes destruction of this vitamin and is not advisable. Some vitamin C (ascorbic acid) is destroyed by the heat and a great deal is dissolved out in the cooking water. The amount of this vitamin in vegetables decreases rapidly on storing and consequently all vegetables should be eaten as fresh as possible.

Green leafy vegetables owe their value in the diet to the ascorbic acid they contain. Because of the ease with which this vitamin is destroyed by heat and dissolved out by water, we should make sure that the cooking reduces the inevitable loss of ascorbic acid to a minimum. This can be done by cooking in a little fat or boiling rapidly in the minimum amount of water for the shortest possible time.

In the first method, sufficient fat to cover the bottom is melted in a saucepan. When the fat is hot, but not smoking, the vegetables are added and the lid placed on the saucepan. The vegetables are cooked gently until tender and served with the liquid in the pan.

In boiling, the vegetables should first be thoroughly washed and soaked as little as possible in salted water. Root vegetables should be sliced and green vegetables shredded in order to reduce the time of cooking. Only sufficient water to prevent burning should be used and salt added to it. The pan should have a tightly fitting lid so that the vegetables are "steam-boiled." The boiling should be for as short a time as possible and the pan should be given an occasional shake. The cooking liquor should be used for soups, stews and gravies.

Root vegetables can be cooked by either of these two methods, and there is the same need to reduce the cooking time to a minimum. Potatoes, beetroot and onions can be baked in the oven. Potatoes can be fried in deep fat and root vegetables in shallow fat. It is worth while baking, and even boiling, potatoes unpeeled since the skin helps to prevent loss of ascorbic acid.

Steaming is not recommended as a method of cooking vegetables. Because it is a slow method it results in very considerable loss of ascorbic acid. Finally, cooked vegetables should never be kept hot for long periods before serving. The destruction of ascorbic acid is very rapid under such conditions.

6. Cereals

Cereals are improved in flavour and made more digestible by the softening of their cellulose and the bursting and gelatinisation of their starch grains during cooking. Rice, tapioca and sago can be baked in a slow oven (120–175° C) with milk and sugar to form milk puddings. Because of the large amount of cellulose, oatmeal should be soaked overnight and boiled for 15–20 minutes next day after the addition of salt.

BREADMAKING

Bread may be described as the product formed by baking a mixture of flour, water and salt which is made porous by the use of yeast or some other means of aeration. By whatever method the bread is aerated it is made lighter and spongier in texture and its attractiveness and digestibility very considerably increased. If we compare the sodden "damper" baked by the squatter in the ashes of his camp fire, ship's biscuits or the "hard tack" of the army with well-made bread we can easily realise the advantages obtained by aeration.

Methods of Aeration

(1) Leaven

The earliest method of aeration consisted in leaving a small portion of dough from one baking to the next. This left-over dough or leaven was quickly infected with micro-organisms from the dust of the air and when mixed with the next batch of dough contained sufficient yeast cells to lighten or leaven it. The bread produced was much inferior to a modern one but was, no doubt, superior to the more primitive bread made in earlier times by covering a round pasty mass of coarsely ground grain and water with red hot ashes and scraping away the ashes when they became cold.

Bread which has not been aerated is known as unleavened bread and is still eaten by Jews at the Feast of the Passover to commemorate the hurried departure of the Israelites from Egypt. Except for this ceremonial use, modern bread is aerated, at any rate in civilised countries.

Modern methods of aeration can be divided into three main types —mechanical, chemical and fermentation.

(2) Mechanical

Aerated bread is made by placing flour with the necessary salt in a strong iron vessel fitted with a mechanical stirrer. Water saturated with carbon dioxide under pressure (similar to soda water) is then added and thoroughly incorporated with the flour by the mechanical stirrer. The dough is eventually forced out of the iron vessel by the pressure of the gas, moulded into loaves and quickly transferred to the oven. The expansion of the gas by the heat of the oven produces the spongy texture of aerated bread.

(3) The use of Sodium Bicarbonate
As explained on page 148, sodium bicarbonate can be used to make bread, but because of the residue of sodium carbonate it is not used on its own. It can, however, be used in combination with buttermilk or sour milk. 1 kg of flour is used with 10 g of bicarbonate of soda and about 600 ml of buttermilk. The product has a characteristic taste and colour.

(4) Baking Powders
Commercial baking powders can be used to make bread. 30 g of baking powder will raise 1 kg of flour.

(5) Fermentation
This involves the use of yeast which will produce carbon dioxide or leaven the flour. One kilo of flour is used with 20 g of yeast and 15 g salt.

The Baking of Bread

The primary ingredients of bread are flour, yeast, water and salt. Other ingredients are usually added such as milk, fat and sugar.

The flour is first of all weighed out and transferred to an earthenware bowl which has previously been warmed. An earthenware bowl is best because it is a bad conductor of heat and it is warmed because yeast ferments best when warm. The salt is next mixed thoroughly into the flour. The salt gives flavour to the bread, strengthens the gluten and acts as a yeast food. The thorough mixing of the salt with the flour is necessary to prevent too great a concentration coming into contact with the yeast and poisoning it. One kg of flour requires two teaspoonfuls of salt to produce the necessary flavour and stabilisation of the gluten. The required amount of yeast is now weighed out (20 g to 1 kg of flour) and mixed with warm water to which a little sugar may be added. The use of warm water is needed to make the yeast more active. Generally speaking the temperature of the water should be between 32°C and 38°C. The object is to produce a dough temperature of about 28°C and the water is cooled slightly when it is mixed with the colder flour. Yeast ferments best at a temperature of 28° C.

A hollow is next made in the flour into which the mixture of warm water, yeast and sugar is poured until sufficient is added to convert the flour into dough. The dough is then thoroughly kneaded to ensure an intimate mixing of all the ingredients and complete absorption of water by the gluten. The bowl is afterwards covered with a cloth to prevent contact with draughts and consequent chilling of the yeast and placed in a warm place to rise or "prove." The yeast ferments the added sugar and by means of its enzymes converts some of the starch of the flour into sugar as well. The carbon dioxide bubbles formed in this way are held inside the dough by the elastic gluten and the dough rises to about double its original bulk in some one and a half hours. It is then turned on a board previously dusted with dry flour to prevent the dough sticking to the board or the hands. Pieces of the dough are cut off and moulded into the required size and shape.

If tins are to be used they should have been warmed and greased. The warming will prevent the dough being chilled and the greasing will make it easy to remove the bread from the tin after baking. The tins should be about half full. Because the dough is greatly distended by the carbon dioxide gas and the gluten under a great strain, the dough should be very carefully handled at this stage.

After placing in the tins the dough is again lightly kneaded to bring the yeast cells into contact with fresh food supplies and again placed in a warm place to rise still further. This second proving gives the dough a chance to recover from the handling to which it has been subjected, which, no matter how carefully carried out, results in some loss of gas and dropping of the dough. When the dough has risen to the tops of the tins they are placed in the oven to bake. The normal temperature for bread is 200–230° C and the time for baking about fifty minutes.

For the first few minutes in the oven the higher temperature results in increased yeast activity and expansion of the gas bubbles and the dough rises rapidly above the top of the tin ("oven spring"). After ten or fifteen minutes the temperature becomes too high for the yeast and it is killed. All fermentation is thus stopped and the loaf is sterilised. The gluten is coagulated and the loaf "set" and fixed in shape even though the carbon dioxide escapes. The alcohol formed by the yeast is driven out by the heat and a good deal of the water of the dough converted into steam. The starch cells are burst and gelatinised, particularly those near the outside of the loaf, because of the greater heat. The outside layers of the loaf are dried and converted into a crust in which some of the starch is changed into dextrin and even sugar and caramel.

When withdrawn from the oven, the loaf cools and the solid crust contracts with the formation of small cracks through which steam can escape from the loaf.

The use of milk or fat in breadmaking has a considerable influence on the appearance, flavour and keeping qualities of the bread apart from the obvious increase in food value. The bread has a smoother texture, a softer crumb and a glossier crust and does not go stale quickly.

Bread is one of our most important foods. In the amounts normally eaten it provides us with something like one-fifth of our kcals and one-fifth of our proteins. In addition, bread is an excellent source of thiamine, iron, nicotinic acid and calcium. Its starch provides our main source of carbohydrate. It is a cheap and palatable food. It lacks fat, but this is made up for by our eating it with butter or margarine. Its large amount of carbohydrate makes it an excellent food to be eaten along with foods rich in animal protein and fat, e.g., cheese, eggs, meat and fish, which supplement its vegetable protein.

CAKES

The primary ingredients of the various types of cakes are flour, sugar, eggs, fat and fruit.

The flour used for cake making should be a "soft" flour, i.e., it should not contain too much gluten. A "strong" flour is apt to make the cake go dry quickly when it is cut and exposed to the air. Soft flour gives a softer mixing which rises evenly when baked and is less likely to rise too much in the centre.

Sugar improves the flavour and food value of a cake. It also improves its texture and appearance and helps to keep it moist. Too little sugar is likely to result in a harsh crumb while too much sugar will weaken the gluten and so cause the cake to sink in the middle during baking. The best type of sugar to use is castor because it easily dissolves and creams well. Coarse grained granulated sugar may not be completely dissolved and so cause specks in the cake during baking. The amount of sugar used should be between one-fifth and one-quarter of the weight of the other ingredients, excluding the fruit.

Many types of fat are used in cake-making but the best is undoubtedly butter because of its superior flavour and because it creams up readily and lightly. The fat forms a film round the particles of starch and gluten in the flour thus preventing them sticking together and enabling them to expand more easily when baked. The mixture becomes more friable or "short" so that the cake crumbles readily in the mouth.

Not only is the food value and texture of the cake improved by the use of fat but it also retains its moisture for a much longer period and consequently does not go stale and dry as quickly as would otherwise be the case.

Eggs are used in cakes as aerating, enriching, moistening and colouring agents. An egg should aerate its own weight of flour and in rich cakes sufficient eggs should be used to make the use of baking powder unnecessary. It is the white of the egg which acts as the aerator. The yolk increases the food value of the cake, improves its colour and supplies additional fat to act as shortening. If sufficient eggs are used for aeration there will be sufficient for moistening the mixture. Otherwise, milk will be needed as an additional moistening agent.

Fruit makes a cake more attractive in appearance and taste. Only the best quality fruit should be used and care taken to so balance the ingredients of the cake as to allow the mixture to support the fruit. Too soft a mixture allows the cherries or other fruit to sink to the bottom and so spoil the texture. The syrup should be washed off cherries and the cherries dried again before using and rubbed in flour. This prevents the syrup from melting during baking and the cherries dropping as the syrup runs down the cake.

Proportions of Ingredients

The balancing of the ingredients is a most important factor in successful cake-making. Below are given a few examples showing the usual proportions of various ingredients. The proportions are by weight—an egg is taken as weighing between 50–60 g.

Type of cake	*Flour*	*Sugar*	*Eggs*	*Butter*	*Fruit*	*B.P.*	*Milk*
Plain cake ..	1	½	¼	½	½	*	*
Cherry cake ..	1	1	1	1	¾	—	—
Rich cake ..	1½	1	1	1	1	*	*
Birthday cake ..	1½	1	1½	1	3	—	—
Christmas cake ..	1½	1	1½	1	4	—	—
Wedding cake ..	1	1	1	1	4	—	—

* As necessary.

From an examination of these proportions the following points should be clear:

1. The weight of sugar should not be more than the weight of flour but should be between one-fifth and one-quarter of the weight of all the ingredients, except the fruit.
2. The weight of eggs should be about equal to the weight of the flour; where this is not the case, e.g., plain cakes, baking powder is necessary for aeration and milk for mixing.
3. The weight of eggs should not be more than one and a half times the weight of the butter.

It is an interesting exercise to compare these proportions with the recipes given in your cookery book. Here are three examples.
1. Plain Fruit Cake Recipe

Flour	Sugar	Eggs	Butter	Fruit	B.P.	Milk
225 g	85 g	55 g	85 g	85 g	1 tsp	160ml (approx.)

We see that:

(*a*) The weight of sugar is less than the weight of flour and also less than one-fifth of the weight of all the ingredients, except the fruit.
(*b*) The weight of eggs is less than the weight of flour so that baking powder and milk are needed for aeration and mixing.
(*c*) The weight of eggs is less than the weight of butter.

2. Moderately Rich Cake Recipe

Flour	Sugar	Eggs	Butter	Fruit	B.P.	Milk
225 g	120 g	120 g	120 g	170 g	½ tsp	If necessary

Again we see that:

(*a*) The weight of sugar is less than the weight of flour but is now equal to one-fifth of the weight of all the ingredients, except the fruit.
(*b*) The weight of eggs is less than the weight of flour but twice as great as in the previous recipe so less baking powder and milk are necessary.
(*c*) The weight of eggs is equal to the weight of butter.

3. Rich Fruit Cake Recipe

Flour	Sugar	Eggs	Butter	Fruit	B.P.	Milk
225 g	170 g	225 g	170 g	225 g	None	None

Here we see that:

(*a*) The weight of sugar is less than the weight of the flour and between one-fifth and one-quarter of the weight of all the ingredients, except the fruit.
(*b*) The weight of eggs is equal to the weight of flour so that baking powder is unnecessary for aeration and milk unnecessary for mixing.
(*c*) The weight of eggs is greater than the weight of butter.

Cake-making Methods
1. Plain Cakes
The flour is sifted in a dry basin and salt and baking powder added. The fat is rubbed into the flour with the tips of the fingers until the mixture looks like fine bread crumbs. The sugar, fruit and other dry ingredients are next added and well mixed. The eggs are well beaten and poured into the mixture. If any milk is necessary it should now be stirred in gradually until the right consistency is obtained. If tins are to be used the mixture should be soft enough to drop from a spoon. If to be baked on a baking sheet the mixture should be stiff enough to be handled and moulded into shape. Baking should be done in a moderately hot oven (200–230° C).

2. Rich Cakes
The larger proportion of fat and sugar in rich cakes makes it necessary to adopt a different method of mixing from that used in plain cakes. The fat and sugar are creamed together very thoroughly by first softening the fat slightly and then beating in the sugar until the mixture is smooth, light and fluffy and looks like whipped cream. The eggs are beaten separately until thick and then stirred into the creamed mixture. The flour and baking powder are now added after being sifted. If any milk is necessary to produce the right consistency it should be added at this stage. The consistency should be thick but soft enough to pour from the mixing bowl into the tin. All the ingredients are stirred in with a circular motion until smoothly blended. Last of all, the fruit is added and stirred in gently.

The cake tins are greased and lined with greaseproof paper to prevent burning. The tins are filled about two-thirds full to allow for rising and a depression made in the middle so that the cake will be flat when risen. The cakes are baked in a moderate oven (175–200° C)—the richer the cake the cooler the oven. When the cakes are baked they will shrink slightly from the sides of the tins and a steel knitting needle pushed into them will come out clean without any unbaked cake sticking to it. The cakes should be allowed to cool for a few minutes before removing from the tins and then carefully placed on a wire cake tray to allow steam to escape from the bottom as well as the top and sides. When perfectly cool, the cakes should be placed in dry airtight tins. Large rich cakes should be wrapped in greaseproof paper.

Cake Faults

A perfect cake should have a smooth top and be baked an even brown all round, above and below. It should be well-risen with the top slightly rounded but not dome-shaped or cracked. Finally it should have a smooth even texture with no large holes or tunnels. The common faults and their possible causes are given below.

1. Cake sinking in the middle during or after baking:
(*a*) Using too much baking powder.
(*b*) Too much butter and sugar in proportion to flour.
(*c*) Too cool an oven.
(*d*) Moving the cake before it is set.

2. Fruit sinking to the bottom:
(*a*) Mixture too soft.
(*b*) Damp fruit.
(*c*) Syrup in cherries, or cherries not properly dried after washing.
(*d*) Too much aerating agent.
(*e*) Opening the oven door before the cake is set.

3. Cake cracking during baking:
(*a*) Lack of steam in the oven.
(*b*) Tins not sufficiently lined.
(*c*) Opening the oven door before the cake is set.

4. A dry cake which goes stale quickly:
(*a*) Too cool an oven and too long baking time.
(*b*) Too stiff a mixture.
(*c*) The use of too much baking powder.
(*d*) Too little fat, sugar and eggs.

5. Open texture:
(*a*) Too much baking powder.
(*b*) Too cool an oven.

(*c*) Insufficient creaming of fat and sugar.
(*d*) Careless mixing.

6. Tunnels in cake:
(*a*) Too hot an oven.
(*b*) Too much baking powder.
(*c*) Mixing the ingredients too much after adding the flour.

7. Cake too heavy:
(*a*) Too large a proportion of fat.
(*b*) Mixing the ingredients too long after adding the flour.
(*c*) Too much liquid.
(*d*) Baking at too low a temperature or not baking long enough.

SPONGES

Sponge mixtures are similar to cake mixtures except that they contain flour, sugar, eggs and flavouring only. The same principles are involved in both mixing and baking.

PASTRY

Pastry is a mixture of flour and fat which gives a crisp and slightly risen article. It is used for giving a case or covering for both sweet and savoury mixtures. The flour used should be dry and of good quality. Butter, lard, dripping, margarine, suet or mixtures of these fats may be used as shortening. Baking powder or self-raising flour is only necessary when the proportion of fat is less than half that of the flour.

There are a number of different types of pastry according to the method used for mixing the fat and the flour, e.g.:

Short Crust. The fat is rubbed into the flour ($\frac{1}{2}$ fat to flour).

Suet Crust. The suet is chopped or shredded finely and mixed with the flour ($\frac{1}{2}$ fat to flour).

Flaky. The fat is spread over the flour and rolled in ($\frac{3}{4}$ fat to flour).

Rough Puff. The fat is mixed with the flour and water in small pieces and rolled in ($\frac{1}{2}$ fat to flour).

Puff. The fat is enclosed in the paste and rolled in (equal fat and flour).

Raised pie-crust or hot water pastry. The fat is melted with warm milk or water and mixed with the flour ($\frac{1}{4}$ fat to flour).

General Directions

Except in the case of raised pie-crust pastry, cold water should be used for mixing and only sufficient used to bind the flour together. Too much water makes the pastry difficult to handle and the pastry is likely to bake hard. The hands and all utensils used should also be cold and the mixture handled very lightly with the tips of the fingers only in order to prevent the fat from melting, otherwise the pastry will be hard and difficult to make up. As air is the aerating agent the flour should be sifted and the pastry lightly handled. It is most important that the fat should be thoroughly mixed with the flour whichever method is adopted. Unless baking powder is being used, the pastry will be lighter and less likely to shrink when baked if it is allowed to stand for some time in a cool place before baking.

The temperature of the oven is also of great importance in pastry-making. Whatever type is being made the temperature of the oven should be high at the beginning (230–260° C). This is necessary to expand the air bubbles and burst the starch cells quickly so that the melted fat can be quickly absorbed. Too low a temperature causes the fat to melt and run out before sufficient starch cells have been burst to absorb it. Such pastry is tough, greasy, heavy and indigestible. Too hot an oven may cause the gluten to coagulate on the outside and form a thin crust before the entrapped air has had time to expand. Such pastry is hard instead of being crisp and light. If the pastry is to be eaten cold it should be cooled slowly or it will be heavy.

CONVENIENCE FOODS

Convenience foods can be defined as any foods that are prepared in such a way that they are easier for the housewife to use than the original food, or they are made available out of season. This is a very wide definition and includes most of the foods found in our larders. The definition must therefore be narrowed, and for our purposes convenience foods will be taken to mean a prepacked combination of foods or ingredients. The object of convenience foods is to curtail preparation and or cooking times and there is an increasing demand for them.

Because of the increasing demand it is important that the differences in food values between the convenience foods and those prepared in the home is fully recognised.

Convenience foods can be divided into three groups:

packet foods
tinned foods
frozen foods

Packet foods. Packet foods are basically of two types:

(*a*) Raw dry ingredients are mixed together and need only the addition of water, milk or egg, followed by normal cooking, e.g. cake mixes.
(*b*) Pre-cooked ingredients which are then air-dried, freeze-dried or accelerated freeze dried. These need reconstituting with water and heating, e.g., soups.

The nutrient value of packet mixes will generally be lower than that of the equivalent food prepared at home with fresh ingredients. The differences may include the following:

(1) The flour may not be fortified.
(2) The dried milk may be fat-free and therefore deficient in milk fats and fat-soluble vitamins.
(3) The fats are likely to be pure fats and will not contain the vitamins A and D present in butter and margarine.
(4) The egg equivalent may be a synthetic raising agent and therefore lacking all the nutrients present in eggs.
(5) The meat may be pre-cooked, shredded, mixed with soya flour and made into a block which is sliced and then dried.
(6) Synthetic flavourings may give the impression that a food is present which is not.
(7) The effects of drying on the nutrient value of foods are described in Chapter 15.

Tinned foods
(*a*) Single foods, e.g. fruit.
(*b*) Complex foods, e.g. stew.
(*c*) Combination tins with different foods in each part of the tin.

The nutrient value of correctly canned foods closely approximates to that of the correctly cooked fresh foods (see Chapter 16). Generally fresh ingredients will not necessarily be the same as those used by the housewife. In particular the flour may not be fortified, egg-substitutes may be used and the fat may not contain vitamins A and D.

Frozen foods

(*a*) Single foods prepared for cooking, e.g. fish fingers.
(*b*) Complex dishes prepared for re-heating, e.g. shepherds pie.
(*c*) Complex dishes prepared and ready to eat, e.g. mousse, cakes, ice-cream.

The nutritive value of all fresh foods when frozen correctly is as high as that of the fresh food. But it cannot be assumed that in the more elaborate dishes the manufacturer will use the same ingredients as would be used in the home, and the nutritive value may be very different.

17 Food Hygiene

FOOD POISONING

We have seen that foods putrefy and decay because of the action upon them of micro-organisms such as bacteria, yeasts and moulds. While the majority of these micro-organisms do no more than lead to the waste of valuable food, there are some which can cause serious outbreaks of food poisoning and disease.

Most cases of food poisoning in this country are caused by three species of bacteria. They are bacteria of the Salmonella group, the staphylococcal group and some other species including clostridium welchii and clostridium botulinum. In addition, pathogenic (disease-carrying) bacteria may find their way into food through the agency of human disease carriers handling the food. Typhoid fever, scarlet fever, undulant fever, tuberculosis and diphtheria have all been known to spread in this way, particularly in milk, drinking water, and fresh or made-up meat. Oysters have been known to cause typhoid fever when the oyster beds have been polluted with sewage water. Steps are now taken to prevent this. Flies, cockroaches and crickets are notorious as conveyors of putrefactive and pathogenic bacteria, and rats and mice have also been held accountable for the infection of foods. Certain animal parasites, e.g. tapeworm, round worm and trichina, may be found in meat.

"Food poisoning" can also be caused by the presence of harmful chemicals in food. Included in the list are the metals lead, zinc and antimony, as well as more complex substances such as pesticides, and substances added as flavourings or dyes.

BACTERIAL FOOD POISONING

The bacteria that cause food poisoning may either themselves infect the person or may cause symptoms as a result of the toxins that they have manufactured.

The infection type of food poisoning takes longer before the symptoms show, and is usually a more severe and more prolonged type of poisoning than that caused by the toxins. Usually with the toxin type of food poisoning, the body's reaction is swift, but after the toxins have been got rid of by sickness and diarrhoea there is a quick recovery. The exception to this is the poisoning by the toxins of clostridium botulinum, which is so severe that it causes damage to the nervous system and often results in death.

The staphylococcal bacteria live in the nose and mouth and on the skin of many people, where they do no positive harm and one is unaware of their presence. They get into the food either directly from the hands or mouth, or indirectly from, for example, a licked spoon, or as a result of picking the nose or handling a soiled handkerchief. Since one is not aware that they are there and some handling of food is inevitable, the only way of minimising infection is to make sure that hands and nails are washed clean, cuts are covered and bad habits eliminated.

Poisoning from staphylococcal toxins shows itself in about 2–3 hours and rarely lasts more than 12 hours.

Salmonella bacteria can often be found in the bowels of man and animals. They get on to food directly if the food is in contact with the faeces of animals, as is likely if rats, mice or flies can wander freely over food, utensils or preparation surfaces. But the usual way for them to be spread to food is as a result of somebody not washing their hands after having been to the toilet. It should be realised that toilet paper is porous and bacteria can readily pass through to the hands. Inanimate objects such as towels, door handles, W.C. equipment, crockery and cutlery may serve as intermediate objects in the transfer of infection from person to person, or from person to food.

Duck eggs may be contaminated with salmonella bacteria when they are laid, and for this reason all duck eggs must be very thoroughly cooked to ensure the destruction of all the salmonella bacteria. No duck eggs should ever be eaten "soft-boiled," nor used in soufflés, omelettes or other similar dishes.

The food poisoning is caused by the salmonella bacteria themselves, and the symptoms—diarrhoea and sickness—do not appear for 12–24 hours after eating the food and may go on for 8 days.

Clostridium welchii is commonly present in small numbers on meat and is probably derived from the bowel contents of the animal. It is destroyed during the thorough cooking of meat, but meat is sometimes not thoroughly cooked. Clostridium welchii causes fairly mild sickness and diarrhoea.

Botulism or food poisoning by clostridium botulinum is very rare and usually fatal. The spores occur in soil and dust, and occasionally find their way into made-up foods, such as sausages and meat pies, and canned goods such as vegetables. The bacteria live without oxygen and produce their toxins in the interior of the food itself, which may not be sufficiently altered in appearance, smell or taste for its infection to be noticeable. The toxin is destroyed by the temperature of ordinary cooking, but the spores are more resistant and are not killed until the temperature reaches 121° C.

Although one takes all possible precautions to prevent bacteria contaminating food, it is not possible to prevent it entirely. Food poisoning will *not* result from eating lightly contaminated food. It will only result from a heavy contamination and usually this means that a light infection is given both the time and the conditions necessary to build up into a heavy contamination.

Bacteria multiply by simple division into two, and this occurs roughly every twenty minutes at suitable temperatures and in suitable media such as meatstuffs, milk and egg dishes. The most suitable temperature for growth is similar to that of the human body. Consequently, food poisoning is commonest in the summer months. Winter outbreaks are usually associated with high kitchen or larder temperatures. At 4° C, the temperature of the average domestic refrigerator, there is no multiplication of bacteria although they do not necessarily die. At temperatures above 45° C, growth is similarly retarded. However, if contaminated food is kept at temperatures between these two extremes, the bacteria will grow and rapidly multiply. Theoretically, one bacterium will form two million in seven hours, but in fact the rate is not quite as high as this; nevertheless, the speed at which high populations of bacteria can develop is easily seen and hence the importance of correct storage for the minimum length of time.

Normally cooking will destroy bacteria and much of the toxins too, but certain types of bacteria are able to develop spores when conditions are unfavourable for normal growth and multiplication, and these spores are much more resistant to high temperatures. When conditions become favourable again the spores revert to the vegetable cell form and multiply rapidly. Let us suppose that a meat dish or a meat gravy is contaminated by a particular food-poisoning, spore-forming bacterium. Ordinary cooking would destroy the vegetable cell forms, but the spores would survive. If the food were eaten at once, the spores would have no opportunity to develop and no harm would be done. The same would be true if the food were quickly cooled and placed in the refrigerator. On the other hand, if such a food were left in a warm kitchen until the following day, the spores might develop into cells which would rapidly multiply. The food might become heavily contaminated and be capable of causing food poisoning.

FOOD HYGIENE

The preceding paragraphs make obvious the need for constant vigilance and strict observation of hygiene practices.

1. Personal Hygiene

Personal hygiene is of first importance so that bacteria from the nose, throat, bowels and skin may not linger on the hands and inadvertently be transferred to foodstuffs. Much of the danger can be eliminated by thorough washing of the hands before touching food, care of the nails and control over such bad habits as touching the nose and licking the fingers. All members of the family should wash their hands before sitting down to meals, and after using the W.C. Any exposed sore or scratch, particularly on hands or arms, should be covered with a waterproof dressing, and a handkerchief should always be held over nose and mouth when coughing or sneezing.

2. Food Handling

In fact, the golden rule is to handle food as little as possible! All food should be kept clean, cool and covered, and special care should be taken in the handling of meat and fish foods which are re-heated, processed or made-up, such as brawn, pies, sausage meat, rissoles, pressed beef, soups and stews. Such foods should be eaten as soon as possible after preparation. Small numbers of pathogenic organisms with which the food might be infected would probably be harmless if eaten shortly after cooking, but will become highly dangerous if kept warm for several hours and allowed to multiply. Puddings, synthetic cream, cream, milk, duck eggs and dried eggs can also be dangerously contaminated.

3. The Cooking of Food

All foods should be kept cool until cooked, cooked thoroughly and eaten immediately after cooking or cooled down at once and kept cool until used.

Cooked food should never be left to cool in a humid kitchen or in a warm oven. Stock should be made from fresh ingredients every day, kept boiling throughout the period of use and discarded at the end of the day.

If food has to be prepared the day before it is to be eaten, it should be cooled as quickly as possible and then placed in a refrigerator or a cool larder.

Food that has to be re-heated should be brought to boiling point before serving and sufficient time allowed to ensure that the *whole* of it reaches boiling point.

4. The Storage of Food

The correct storage of food is vitally important, as it serves the dual functions of preventing contamination and providing conditions unsuitable for the multiplication of bacteria.

All food should be stored so that animals and insects cannot reach it.

Meat, fish, milk and food with gelatine or cream in it must be kept as cool as possible.

More details of the correct design and use of larders and refrigerators will be found in Chapter 19. It is impossible to overemphasise the importance of correct storage for the minimum length of time, as this will greatly reduce the incidence of food poisoning.

5. Kitchen Hygiene

Kitchen hygiene is also of vital importance. All crockery and utensils must be thoroughly washed and rinsed. With a double sink and plenty of hot water at about 85° C, crockery and utensils can be sterilised and will dry quickly without a drying cloth.

If drying cloths must be used they should be changed frequently and washed daily. Otherwise they can harbour millions of bacteria. Dish cloths must also be kept scrupulously clean.

All working surfaces should be impervious to liquids and without open cracks and should be kept scrupulously clean, as should all fittings, walls and floor.

The housewife should always wear a clean overall when handling and cooking food.

Domestic animals should not be allowed in rooms where food is stored, prepared, or cooked.

Waste food should be kept in bins with closely fitting lids until disposed of. Dustbins should be kept in good order with a firmly fitting lid.

Flies should be destroyed and ventilators of larders covered with wire mesh screens. Crevices round pipes, and cracks or faulty joints in walls, should be sealed to deny access to cockroaches.

Rats and mice should be exterminated.

6. General Hygiene

Public health authorities employ inspectors to examine meat and other foods, and places where food is prepared and sold, in order to prevent the sale of foods unfit for human consumption. The utmost cleanliness is essential in all abattoirs, bakeries, food factories, markets, shops, hotels, restaurants and, not least, the home, to prevent infection of food by people, rats, mice, flies, cockroaches and crickets.

Great advances have been made in our methods of handling food at all stages, but there is still room for further improvements and an informed public opinion can do much to bring them about. As citizens we have the protection of legislation and the public servants to enforce it; as individuals we can buy or eat our food in establishments with a reputation for cleanliness and we can carry out clean food practices in our own homes.

Pathogenic bacteria usually get into food via contaminated water, but it is also possible for a person to carry the germs of certain diseases without realising that they are there. A "carrier" has always had the disease, although sometimes the attack is very mild; he then, to all appearances, recovers from the disease; but in fact, he continues to harbour the bacteria. If such a carrier is not very careful about hygiene and then handles food or food containers, he will pass the infection on to others. It is, therefore, essential that carriers should be identified and isolated until the infection has been eliminated.

The use of clean water for all processes concerned with the production and handling of food is absolutely essential if pathogenic bacteria are not to infect food; the greatest care in rigidly observing all the hygiene measures described in the previous section is also essential.

METAL POISONING

The most common metal poisoning is from lead, but food is sometimes contaminated by zinc or antimony. This is usually the result of storing acid foods, e.g. fruit salad or fruit juices, in zinc or poor quality enamelled containers. To avoid risk of these metals being dissolved into the food, it is essential not to use such containers.

PART FOUR

18 The Kitchen

The average housewife spends 75% of her working time in the kitchen, and it is therefore essential to consider with great care the design, the materials used in the construction of the kitchen and the choice of both the large equipment such as cookers and the smaller utensils.

Before doing this, however, it is useful to consider what activities are likely to go on within the kitchen. To a certain extent these activities will be influenced by the size and age of the family, but will always include food storage, preparation, cooking and washing up; for most families the clothes washing will also be done in the kitchen, and probably the ironing. Many families like to eat in the kitchen, and young children like to follow their mothers as they work, so that if possible there should be sufficient room for them to be in the kitchen at the same time as their mothers. The kitchen is thus likely to be needed as a store room, work room for preparation of meals and laundering, and also for some of the social activities of the home. No other room has so many functions to fulfil, and with growing realisation of its importance has grown an increasing emphasis on careful design, fittings, and an increase in size.

When designing the room it is essential to consider a variety of aspects including its efficiency as a centre for its activities, its safety and the comfort with which it may be used.

Influencing *efficiency* will be:— the size and shape of the room, the layout of the equipment, the materials used for floor, walls and ceiling, and the lighting, ventilation and heating.

Safety is also a factor that must be considered in a room where so much complex equipment is being used, and where sources of intense heat, and water, and electricity are all likely to be present. The danger of accidents from falling, and from knocking into open cupboard doors, must also be considered. Kitchen *hygiene* is discussed in Chapter 17.

The *comfort* of the kitchen is the third factor that must be considered; to a large extent one can assume that if the features of design necessary to produce an efficient and safe room are incorporated then the room will be a comfortable one to use, and yet more is needed to produce a comfortable room than the factors which could lead to a room of clinical sterility and efficiency. It is therefore necessary to consider such aspects as the use of colour and texture in adding comfort to the kitchen.

SIZE AND SHAPE OF THE KITCHEN

Ideally a kitchen should be large enough (i) for the basic work of food storage, preparation, cooking and washing up to be carried out in it; (ii) for laundering to be done in it—unless of course separate laundry facilities are provided; (iii) to allow the family to eat there if they wish to do so; (iv) for small children to play there without getting in the way. The Dept of the Environment recommendations for the space needed for these basic activities can be found in *Space in the Home*, published by H.M. Stationery Office.

Unfortunately many people have kitchens that fall far below these ideals, and before considering the actual arrangement of the kitchen furniture, certain basic principles must be borne in mind. First, the equipment must not be placed so that the doorways are blocked, and it may be useful to consider re-hanging the doors or the use of sliding or folding doors if there is any risk of the doors causing accidents. The insertion of toughened glass panels into a previously solid door may also help to prevent accidents. Secondly, there must be sufficient space for people to move safely around in the room, and thirdly the working areas must be adequately lit.

Adequate drainage and water supply must be available and a source of running hot water is also now an accepted minimum standard. Gas may be installed or only electricity. The Dept of the Environment recommends a minimum of four electric socket outlets, and if an electric cooker is used this will need to have its own socket outlet and correct wiring.

Sometimes it is possible to alter the kitchen fairly easily and at comparatively little cost; thus, for instance, the installation of a new window may greatly improve a room; knocking down a wall between a kitchen and larder or kitchen and scullery may also be fairly simple ways of making the room larger and more efficient.

The consideration of all these factors before finally deciding on the actual layout of equipment will be of immeasurable benefit.

It is generally accepted that a work sequence of working surface—cooker—working surface—sink—working surface is desirable, and that this sequence should not be interrupted by doors. This sequence gives maximum efficiency and also maximum safety. There are basically two possible ways of arranging this work sequence, depending on whether this part of the room is shaped as a corner or is a passage room (see diagram).

As well as the arrangement of sink and cooker, other important equipment in the kitchen may include washing machine, refrigerator and of course storage space.

The type of washing machine will largely affect its position in the kitchen; those machines that complete the full cycle of washing,

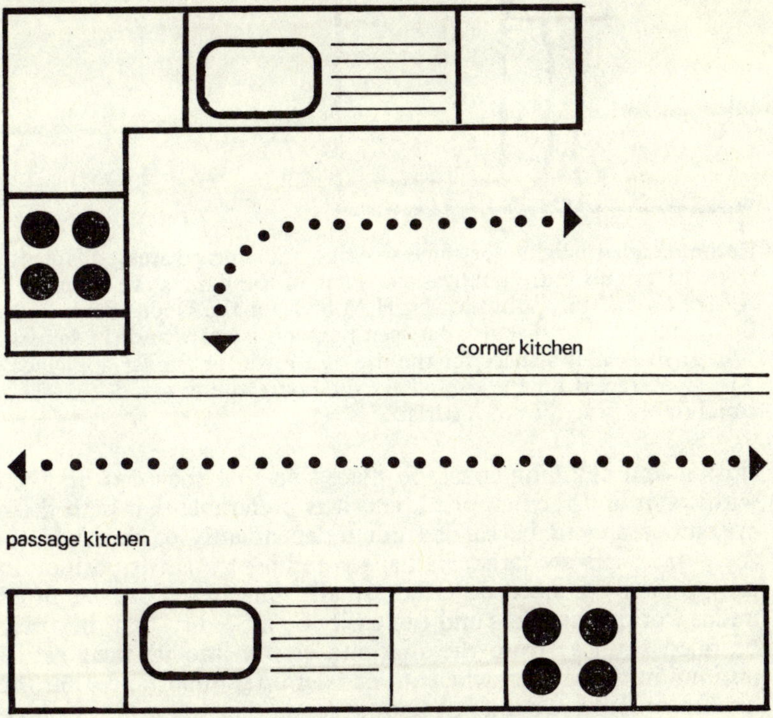

Diagrams of "corner" and "passage" kitchens.

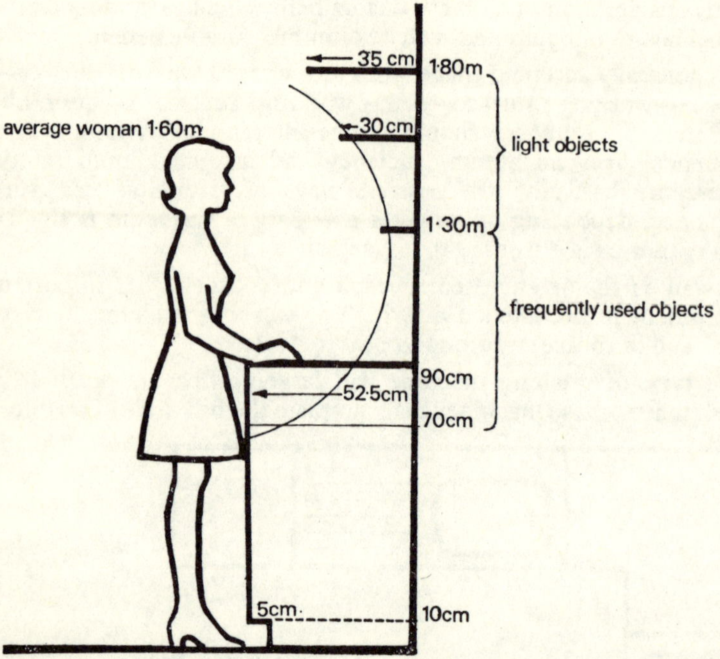

Recommended heights for some working and storage areas, adapted from a Design Centre publication. Some of the figures are from *Space in the Home*, published by H.M.S.O. for the Dept of the Environment. The distance between the work surface and the lowest storage shelf allows space for the use of a mixer or similar appliance. The small recess for the feet allows the housewife to stand comfortably near the work surface.

rinsing and spinning must be placed so that they can be filled with water and then emptied, and it is preferable that both these operations should be carried out independently of the sink. As these machines are large, wall space and a permanent position in the kitchen are needed. Other smaller machines can be fitted under working surfaces and can easily be moved so that they may be filled by hose from the sink and empty into it; their actual position in the kitchen when stored is of little importance, but the kitchen must have sufficient floor space so that when the machine is in use it is still possible to move safely around in the room.

The position of the refrigerator is of importance in terms of convenience in use, and there must be sufficient space for the insertion and removal of food. If possible, it should be near to the food preparation surfaces.

Storage space is extremely important. A ventilated cupboard, or larder, is essential if there is no refrigerator, and further space is needed for the storage of other food, and for cooking and eating utensils. A minimum of 2·3 cubic metres is suggested by the Dept of the Environment in *Homes for Today and Tomorrow.* This storage space will include the cupboards under the sink unit, the larder or food cupboard, and other wall fittings. The exact position of these fittings will be determined by the position of other items in the kitchen, but by the careful arrangement of storage space it is possible to increase the working efficiency of the kitchen. Thus by storing food near the food preparation area, saucepans by the stove and so on, a great deal of unnecessary fetching and carrying may be avoided.

Floor, Walls and Ceiling

The choice of materials suitable for covering the floor, walls and ceiling of a kitchen is probably more difficult than for any other room. For one thing the kitchen which serves as a food preparation room, laundry and possibly also as a living room is used for a greater variety of purposes, but also the conditions that these materials must withstand include not only hard wear, but they must also be easily cleaned and must resist damp, heat and grease.

FLOOR

The floor of the kitchen may be of concrete or in some cases of wood. To cover it, a material must be found that is not only easily cleaned, resistant to damp and is hardwearing, but also one that can withstand considerable weights without being dented, is not affected by grease, does not stain, is not slippery, and is not too cold, nor too hard, for the housewife's feet. Several types of floor covering are available; none of them possesses all the required characteristics, but the following are the most suitable.

Linoleum. This should preferably be inlaid and have a mottled finish (jaspe) so as not to show every mark as a plain linoleum does. Linoleum can be laid over wood, concrete or tiles, provided the surface is not uneven, and is usually more satisfactory when stuck to the floor with adhesive. If the floor is not provided with a damp course the linoleum will eventually rot unless a damp-proof material is placed between it and the floor. Linoleum can be kept clean by washing with a mild detergent, provided it is thoroughly dried afterwards, but the best form of maintenance is polishing with a good wax polish to prevent it from becoming dry and brittle. The use, according to maker's instructions, of a good floor sealer reduces the working of cleaning. If well maintained, linoleum is quiet, resilient and hard wearing, and, unless highly polished, not slippery. It is not a dense, hard material and is indented if very heavy equipment is placed on it; while if it is treated with coarse abrasives or strong alkalis, the surface will be penetrated and the linoleum will disintegrate in time. Linoleum is an absorbent material and any water spilled on it should be wiped off as quickly as possible to prevent rotting, particularly in front of the sink. Linoleum becomes brittle when dry and is thus liable to crack and wear round the cooker.

Stone tiles. Tiles are tough, hard, durable, and resistant to grease, high temperatures and alkalis, but they are expensive. They show every footmark and hence need constant cleaning. Fortunately, washing with a good detergent and a mop or scrubbing brush is all that is required. Apart from their high cost, the main faults of tiles are that they are cold, noisy and tiring to the feet.

Thermoplastic flooring. Thermoplastic floorings are hard-wearing, reasonably quiet and resilient, and not slippery unless wet or highly polished. They are not heat resistant and tend to soften near the cooker. For this reason the cooker should be placed on a stone tiled inset. This type of flooring has a tendency to indentations from heavy objects and is apt to mark badly with such things as rubber heels or Wellington boots. These marks can only be removed with fine steel wool and a little abrasive powder, but this should not be done too frequently or the surface will be permanently roughened. Ordinary cleaning of thermoplastic floors can be done with hot water and a detergent. Ordinary wax polishes containing spirit solvents should not be used as they damage the floor.

Rubber floor coverings, either natural or synthetic, are very resilient and hard wearing, quiet, warm, non-slipping and resistant to abrasion, but they will not withstand excessive heat or strong light. Fat and grease cause deterioration and should be wiped off immediately, or the rubber will become tacky in time. Alkalis and spirit do not affect rubber but turpentine does. For this reason wax polishes containing turpentine should not be used on rubber floors. Washing with hot water and a detergent is the best method of cleaning. Polishing is not really necessary, but if a wax polish is used it should be of the water emulsion type.

Flexible (Polyvinyl Chloride) sheeting. This is fairly hard wearing and is easily cleaned by wiping over with hot water and detergent. It is not slippery when dry, but does become more slippery when wet. It indents with heavy articles of furniture, stains with some grease based stains (e.g. shoe polish) and is marked by the heels of some shoes. After being laid it shrinks somewhat, and the edges of the sheets tend to curl. Some p.v.c. has a felt backing; this increases its resilience but makes it more susceptible to damp and to indentation by heavy objects. It is not really suitable for kitchens. Non-slip granules can be incorporated into the flexible p.v.c. floor coverings, and this greatly improves its non-slip aspect even when it is wet.

WALLS

The walls of the kitchen must be smooth, easily cleaned and resistant to grease and damp. For this reason ordinary wall paper and distemper are not suitable, but a number of other finishes are available.

Paint. The walls can be painted with a heat and damp-resisting paint. The plastic paints, e.g. polyurethane paints, are probably the most suitable yet developed as they give a hard smooth and washable surface.

Tiles. Tiles can be used all over the walls or limited to areas where there is a lot of splashing, for instance behind the sink and adjacent to the cooker. The development of cheap decorative tiles has increased the decorative potential of tiling.

Wallpaper. As it is important that the surface of the wall is washable, only those papers with a truly washable finish are suitable, and for this reason the vinyl papers are ideal and allow great scope for imaginative use of colours and textures in the decor.

CEILING

The best finish for ceilings is a heat and damp and grease-resisting one that is smooth, non-absorbent and easily cleaned, and the best finish is probably given by a simple painted finish, polyurethane paints giving the hardest surfaces. In a kitchen where condensation on the ceiling presents a considerable problem, expanded polystyrene tiles can be used, but these should then be painted so that the surface can be easily cleaned.

LIGHTING

The lighting of the kitchen is extremely important and affects not only the efficient use of the room but also its safety.

So far as is possible, the kitchen, like all other rooms in a house, should be lit by daylight. This means that the windows must be large and that the older type of kitchen whose windows often faced a wall is far from suitable. Probably ideal are windows facing east so that the sun lights the room in the morning but passes round later in the day so that the room does not become too hot. Windows must be of such a type that they can be opened without causing an obstruction in the room, and the kitchen stove should not be so close to the window that the curtains can be blown across the stove.

In kitchens where the windows face south or west, and where the sun may be too strong, the use of blinds will reduce the glare and keep the room cooler, but the cleaning of these blinds can be troublesome and terylene net which is easily washed may prove to be more labour-saving.

Artificial lighting must be so placed that it lights all the working surfaces, the sink and the stove, the light falling on the surface in such a way that the person working is not in her own shadow. This usually means that there must be at least two lights. The adequate lighting of cupboards is also important.

The use of fluorescent lights is advisable as they give an extremely good all-round light and, although expensive to instal, are cheap to run and do not give off much heat. The careful choice of decorative schemes will enhance the lighting effects.

VENTILATION

The ventilation of the kitchen requires careful consideration. Good ventilation reduces the condensation of steam which is so detrimental to the walls, prevents cooking odours penetrating into the rest of the house and keeps the kitchen cool.

Different types of window are available; all have various advantages and disadvantages in terms of actual opening area, space occupied and ease of cleaning. But there are times when it is inconvenient to have a window open but when the kitchen still needs considerable ventilation; for this reason the installation of some kind of ventilating device is extremely useful.

One of the simplest is the disc type in which a small quatrefoil device is inserted into a fixed pane and a spinning disc causes some exchange of air.

Electric extractor fans are more expensive but more efficient. There are two basic types: one is simply an extractor fan which takes air out of the kitchen, the other has a two-way circulation bringing in air from outside as well as removing it.

The installation of a cooker hood with a ventilating shaft leading to the extractor fan is an extension of this principle and ensures that steam, vapourised fat and cooking odours are efficiently removed. Cooker hoods that do not lead to a ventilating shaft do not help in the ventilation but do help to remove grease and cooking odours.

HEATING

The minimum temperature in the working kitchen should be 12° C. In the kitchens where there is a solid fuel stove which gives off sufficient heat to warm the room the problem is usually to ensure that the room can be cooled—especially in the summer. But in kitchens where there is no solid fuel stove it is essential to have some form of heating other than the cooking stove. The heating should preferably be efficient so that it will quickly warm the room, and easily controllable so that the room does not become overheated.

Gas fires need to be installed with a flue and must be adequately guarded to prevent accidents; they do however give instant heat and are easily controlled. They are not normally recommended for a small kitchen because of the difficulty of installation and the danger of people, or clothes, falling into them.

Electric fires must be adequately guarded and only infra-red or panel heaters should be used in a room such as the kitchen where there is the danger of wet hands or clothes coming into contact with the fire.

Radiators, either oil or water filled, are the ideal heating for kitchens as they are safe, easily regulated, easily cleaned and take up little floor room.

Warm air heating can be used for heating a kitchen, but it is important to avoid recirculation of the air from the kitchen as it is likely to spread the odours of cooking round the house.

COLOUR SCHEMES

The choice of colour scheme will be affected by the amount and quality of daylight and the size of the room as well as by personal taste. However, whatever scheme is used, it is essential that one can easily distinguish the edges of the working surfaces and any projecting corners (which should be avoided, of course, if possible). A warm kitchen with a bright aspect will need a cool colour scheme: white, grey, blue or green may well feature in this; a darker, colder room will need warmer colours and white, orange, red and yellow can be used to highlight and warm the room. The use of too many colours should be avoided as it makes a room look small and untidy.

The most permanent features of a kitchen are the working surfaces and the main equipment, e.g. sink and the cooker; the floor coverings, the walls and the woodwork are renewed more frequently. As the permanent features have to be lived with for a long time, it is advisable to think carefully before deciding and to choose a colour that one will not quickly tire of, and that will blend or contrast with a variety of the colours that one may choose for the rest of the kitchen over the years.

Generally, then, it is wise to stick to a basic pale colour for most of the surfaces and to highlight it with vivid touches of bright colour, e.g. in the curtains, in handles and knobs of doors, drawers, etc., and in the wallpaper.

MAJOR ITEMS OF KITCHEN EQUIPMENT

The processes that go on in the kitchen require that there should be storage space for food, china and cooking utensils, working surfaces for the preparation of food, a sink and draining board for washing and washing up and a cooker. Other useful large items include a refrigerator, a washing machine and a dishwasher, considered in Chapter 19. Smaller items of equipment will be considered in Chapter 20.

STORAGE SPACE

The Dept of the Environment suggests a minimum of 2·3 cubic metres for storage of all types in a kitchen; this space will be needed for the storage of cleaning materials, dry goods, perishable foods as well as all the utensils needed during cooking.

19 Large Equipment

SINKS

The sink is usually fixed on an outside wall below a window to reduce plumbing costs and to allow work at the sink to be done in a good light. The wall round the sink should be of some smooth, easily cleaned material, e.g., tiles, enamel or oil paint. The floor immediately beneath the sink should be of some smooth, easily cleaned waterproof material. The height of the sink is usually the same as that of the general kitchen working surfaces, i.e., 900 mm. Ideally, the user should be able to touch the bottom of the sink with the finger-tips without bending. A toe recess should be left below if the sink is fitted with a cupboard underneath.

Stone and fireclay were formerly used for sinks, but these materials are difficult to keep clean and have now been replaced by glazed earthenware, sheet steel finished with vitreous enamel, stainless steel, aluminium, an alloy of nickel and copper known as Monel metal, or plastics. All materials used for sinks should be able to stand up to heavy usage. Glazed earthenware is strong and durable but the vitreous glaze can be broken by a hard blow. Chipping or cracking spoils the appearance of the sink and makes cleaning more difficult.

Sheet steel or cast iron finished with vitreous enamel is durable and easily cleaned and can be colourful. Stainless steel, aluminium or Monel metal sinks are more expensive but very durable and do not chip or corrode. Rough usage will, however, scratch the surface and so spoil the appearance of the sink, particularly if it has a shiny finish. Metal sinks with a matt finish do not show scratches as easily but are more difficult to keep free from grease. Any metal sink is liable to be noisy in use, but this can be reduced by fitting a wooden frame underneath to absorb some of the vibration and so deaden the sound.

Plastic sinks are colourful, quiet in use and resilient enough to reduce breakages of crockery and glassware. They do not chip but, if subjected to rough usage, may stain, scratch or even crack. The length and breadth of the sink will vary according to the size of the kitchen and the amount of work to be done in it, but the depth should never be less than 230 mm. All sinks should be fitted with a rubber plug and chain and the waste pipe should have a grating. All sinks should have an overflow grating and pipe. Double sinks are convenient for the rinsing of objects that have been washed in synthetic detergents. Some sinks can be fitted with waste disposal units.

Even if space is limited it is a great advantage to have a draining board on each side of the sink. They should slope slightly towards the sink and be grooved to enable water to drain away easily, but not so steeply sloped as to allow plates to slide. If not moulded with the sink, they should be easily removable for cleaning and should slightly overlap the sink. The joints with both sink and wall should be greaseproof and waterproof. Wooden draining boards should not be used.

The taps should be correctly placed so that the spouts are at least 300 mm from the inside bottom of the sink. A bucket or large jug can then be conveniently placed inside the sink for filling. The pillar type single tap with one spout for hot and cold water is particularly convenient for the kitchen sink. Since kitchen taps are given very hard use they should be so constructed as to make it easy to renew worn-out washers. Kitchen taps should preferably be of plated metal to reduce cleaning.

A plate rack which holds the crocks firmly and drains them effectively is a useful adjunct to the sink. It is usually made from rustless metal or plastics. It should be easily cleaned and simple in design. It is best fixed above a draining board and should have a detachable tray on which the plates and dishes can drip.

DISHWASHERS

These may be free-standing or built in, and vary in size and complexity. Basically there are two designs: one distributes the water from the base of the machine, the other sprays the water on from rotating jets. Most machines have an automatic cycle of washing and rinsing; some heat the water, others rely on household hot water; some dry the crockery, others don't. All the machines

R

work better with soft water; some machines have to have softened water, others rely on water softeners present in the detergent.

The design of the racks in the machines, the size and the degree of automation are all important points to consider when choosing a machine.

Regular servicing of the machines is essential and running costs are fairly high.

COOKERS

Cookers may be heated by solid fuel, gas, electricity or oil. Modern cookers, whether solid-fuel, gas, electricity or oil heated, are now so efficient and reliable that usually any poor results obtained with them should be put down to the faulty adjustment of the cookers or the housewife's mismanagement of them. Each type of cooker has its own particular advantages and disadvantages and the choice between them becomes largely a question of cost, convenience, services available, and personal preference.

Gas and electric cookers are the most common types in use today with gas still the more popular of the two. There is little difference in the price of gas or electric cookers of similar capacity. Servicing costs should be taken into account. Running costs vary according to local tariffs. Eighteen to twenty units of electricity provide as much heat as one therm of gas and relative costs can be assessed on this basis, but differences in running costs are not likely to be a decisive factor in choosing between the two. Essentially, gas is more convenient for cooking than electricity, because it can be adjusted immediately to almost any required temperature.

By its nature, electricity should be cleaner and safer. But the differences between the two are becoming less and less as electric cookers are made more flexible and gas cookers safer and easier to clean. Thus, personal preference is the main factor in the choice of a modern cooker.

Nowadays cookers have come to be regarded as appliances providing an oven for baking, a hob for boiling, etc. and a compartment for grilling. Usually these are fixed vertically one above the other, because this arrangement takes up least space in the small modern kitchen. Where more floor space is available, horizontal cookers can be used in which the oven and grill are side by side under an overall hob or with the base of the oven level with the base of the hob at its side.

Another development is the unit cooker in which the components are separate and complete in themselves and are built into the kitchen fitments in any position and at any height to suit the user's convenience. In the future, individual heat-controlled cooking apparatus such as saucepans, kettles, frying pans, grills, toasters, pressure cookers and so on may supersede the traditional cooker in the same way as the open fire with its various cooking gadgets was superseded in the past.

Whichever type of cooker is chosen it should be able to operate over a wide range of temperatures and be satisfactory for the cooking of complete meals which include dishes requiring very different temperatures. It should be compact, attractive in appearance, easy to clean, safe in use and free from unpleasant smell. It should be capable of boiling water quickly, toasting bread efficiently, and heating the contents of a pan rapidly or allowing them to simmer gently from the same source. It should be fitted with several heating points which can be used simultaneously and, if necessary, at varying temperatures. The user should be able to bring the cooker into use at a moment's notice without labour in preparation and should be able to turn it off with the minimum loss of heat. The oven should be easy to regulate and provision should be made for warming plates and keeping dishes hot during the process of cooking without using additional fuel.

Specially designed saucepans should not be required, and pots, pans and kettles of various shapes and sizes should be equally efficient in use. Finally, a great deal of bending and stooping should not be needed when the oven is in use.

This is a formidable list of requirements, but the modern cooker meets the majority of them. The least satisfactory feature of the standard modern cooker and one of the most difficult for manufacturers to improve is that of convenience in use. The oven and "waist-level" grill are too low and necessitate constant bending in use, and the hob is rather too high for the majority of women. Hobs should be about 850 mm from the ground *or* installed so that they come into line with the neighbouring working surfaces. The best position for the oven comes somewhere between waist and shoulder level, which eliminates stooping. For easy viewing, the grill should be at eye level, and for easy manipulation at waist level, so a position between the two seems a reasonable compromise. The hob is used very much more than either the oven or the grill and its height is the most important consideration. Perhaps the only really satisfactory solution to this problem of heights is, as previously mentioned, to consider the oven, hob and grill as separate entities and to fix them at heights most convenient to the user, but this would involve increasing the cost.

Cleaning of Ovens

Traditionally ovens are designed to minimise the difficulty of cleaning, but this has had to be done with abrasives. Three recent developments have made the task of cleaning easier.

(1) *Chemical cleansers.* These are strongly caustic. They may be liquid or solid; probably the easiest to apply is the spray, and this can be put on to a hot surface so that the action is extremely fast. Manufacturers' instructions should be carefully followed.

(2) *Special linings.* A variety of finishes may be applied to the inner surfaces of the oven, which help to reduce the residual dirt. They rely on the heat of the oven to vaporise or break down the deposits.

(3) *Auto-clean ovens.* These are only available in electric cookers. They are heavily insulated and after being locked closed the heat within the oven is raised to about 500° C. All the dirt is burnt off and all that is left is a fine ash. The cycle of heating and cooling takes between 2 and 3 hours.

Solid-Fuel Cookers

Solid fuels include the different varieties of coal, such as ordinary bituminous coal and the smokeless Welsh steam coal and anthracite, as well as coke and patent smokeless fuels.

The old-fashioned coal range has largely been superseded by gas, electric or heat-storage cookers, but some people have of necessity to use one. Such ranges take up a lot of space, are very wasteful of fuel and make the room very dirty because of dust and smoke. They entail a great deal of work in keeping them clean and in lighting, stoking and cleaning out. In summer time they make the kitchen uncomfortably hot; on the other hand, they can be used to supply the household with hot water, and warm the room as well as cooking food. Some housewives are quite prepared to put up with the inconvenience and work of the coal range for the sake of a cheerful blaze in the kitchen.

Nowadays there are improved kitchen ranges and combination grates in vitreous enamel which are modern in appearance, much more easily cleaned and burn fuel more economically and with less dirt and smoke.

In addition to the open coal range there are two types of solid-fuel continuously burning cookers. They are the fully insulated heat-storage cooker and the semi-insulated cooker.

In the *heat-storage cooker*, the fuel is burned continuously at the same rate in a fire-box totally enclosed in the centre of the cooker.

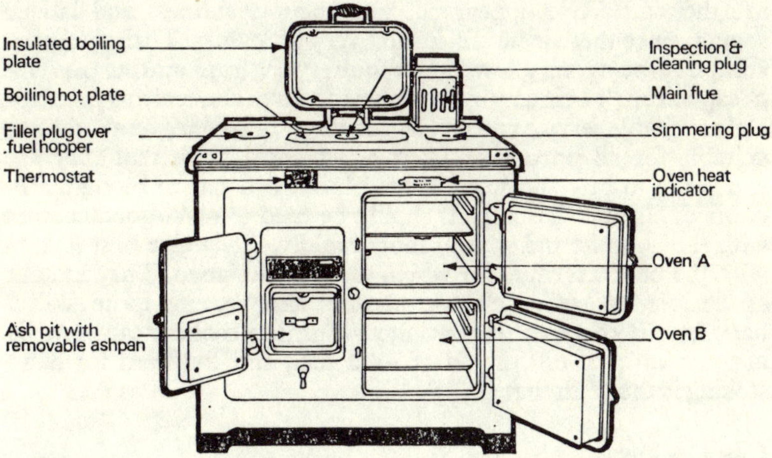

A solid-fuel cooker (the Aga).

Considerable wastage of heat occurs during periods when the ordinary solid-fuel range is not actually in use but in the heat-storage cooker this heat is stored in a heavy iron block above the fire (the hotplate) and in the heavy castings surrounding the ovens. The plate is fitted with an insulated hinged cover to prevent the loss of heat when the hot plate is not in use. The ovens and hot-plate are thus always at working temperatures. A typical design for the ordinary small household has a hot roasting oven on the right-hand side with a temperature of 200–230°C, a medium-heat oven under the fire-door with a temperature of 150–175°C, and a simmering oven with a temperature of about 93°C. Some types have a hot water boiler fitted. The usual fuels for the heat-storage cooker are coke or anthracite.

The *semi-insulated solid-fuel cooker* is cheaper than the heat-storage cooker and more flexible in use but less economical in fuel. With the semi-insulated cooker the rate of combustion of the fuel can be varied by air and damper controls to boost up the fire when cooking. Unlike the heat-storage cooker its fire can be opened and used to warm the kitchen. One type is made in two parts which are built back-to-back in one wall so that the oven half can be in the kitchen and the fire part in the dining room.

The great advantages of the continuous-burning solid-fuel cookers are their attractive appearance and their cleanliness and labour saving, since there is no smoke and very little dust. Their fuel consumption being very low they require very little stoking and are cheap to run. Their continuous burning gives convenient, immediately available service and a balanced range of cooking temperatures suitable for all purposes. Their disadvantages are that they are expensive to buy and need a flue pipe which has to be regularly cleaned. Ground-based pans should be used to make good contact with the hotplate and so heat more rapidly. They give best service with the particular fuel for which they are designed. They are not as flexible as gas or electric cookers and require more skilful handling. Both types of continuous-burning cookers can now be adapted to burn oil instead of solid fuel, and the need for hand stoking is thus eliminated.

Gas Cookers

In gas cookers the heat comes from open flames and the cooking is done by heat which flows round the saucepans or through the oven and then escapes either directly into the air or through suitable vents. Unlike the closed ovens of the solid-fuel, electric or oil types, the gas oven is open below to admit air to burn the gas and consequently convection currents are much stronger.

In recent years great advances have been made in the technical efficiency of the gas cooker. Its vitreous enamel finish gives it an attractive appearance and makes it easy to clean. Insulation of the sides helps to retain the heat, reduces gas consumption and keeps the kitchen cool. The oven thermostatic control makes the gas oven extremely easy to use, corrects for the chilling effect of

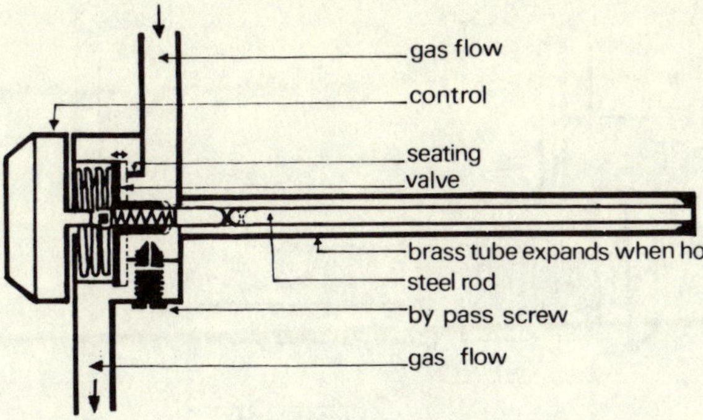

Solid-type gas thermostat. When the gas is burning, the brass tube becomes heated, and as it expands it carries with it the inner steel rod (which expands very little) and brings the valve head closer to its seating, thus reducing the flow of gas. Should the air in the oven cool down, the brass tube becomes less hot, contracts a little and moves the valve slightly away from its seating. This allows more gas to pass to the burner until once again the proper temperature is reached. By courtesy of British Gas.

placing cold food in the oven, cuts down the gas as the food becomes hot and maintains a constant cooking temperature.

A liquid type of thermostat is coming increasingly into use. It consists of a phial connected by capillary tubing to flexible bellows. The phial is filled with liquid which vaporises at a suitable temperature and causes the bellows to expand. This movement is utilised to open or close a gas valve. This liquid type is more flexible than the solid type of thermostat in which the rod and control assembly must of necessity be located together. The phial and control assembly can be located independently because of the flexibility of the capillary tubing. In some gas cookers the phial is located in the flue, thus making the ceiling of the oven free from encumbrance and making an easily cleaned removable top possible. Automatic ignition is now usual on all gas cookers and this makes it possible to provide time-control mechanisms which enable the oven to be pre-set to come on and go off in the housewife's absence.

In the modern gas cooker the oven and hotplate sections are built as separate units, carried in a light structural frame from which

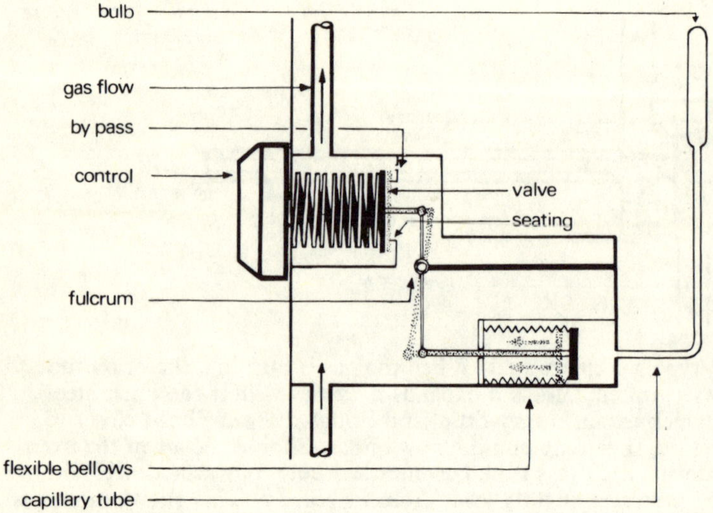

Liquid-type thermostat. The pressure exerted in the sealed system of the heated bulb and the capillary tube is passed to the exterior by a flexible bellows, so as to vary its length by compressing it. This movement is used to operate a lever which is pivoted on a fulcrum and connected to a gas valve at its other end. Thus, as the bulb is heated, the valve is made to move forward to its seating under the action of the spring, and vice versa on cooling. By adjusting the lever position it is possible to pre-set the temperature at which the valve will shut and cut off the flow of gas except for the small safety by-pass. By courtesy of British Gas.

either unit can be withdrawn. The outside casing is easily demountable. Extensive use is made of vitreous enamelled sheet steel, cast iron being used where direct flame contact or very hot gases are encountered, e.g., burners, hotplate pan supports and burner chamber nozzle, and where structural strength is necessary, e.g., the top back plate and the gas rail. New vitreous enamels have been used for the hotplate top and pan supports where heat resistance, corrosion resistance and a smooth finish are important.

The whole oven is designed to economise in gas and to be easily cleaned. The oven shell, which is made in one piece, is secured to the front frame by four insulated bolts. The oven is thus suspended in air. This and the lagging of the oven with a blanket of glass wool covered with aluminium foil reduce the loss of heat by conduction to the frame to a minimum. The oven door beds on a springy strip of metal and the latching works on the cam principle so that when the door is closed the oven is effectively sealed. The oven burners are fixed at the bottom of the oven along the back.

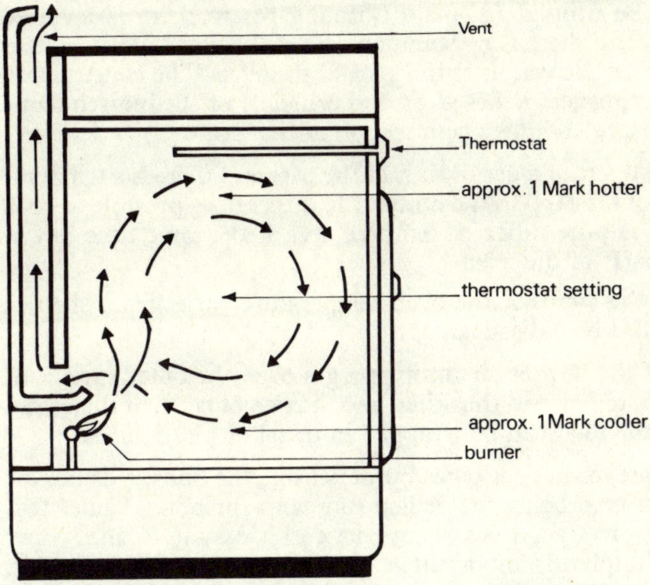

The working of the gas cooker.
The drawing shows the side view of a popular type gas cooker, with the gas pipes omitted. When the burner is lighted the heat rises as shown by arrows, causes the thermostat to expand (automatically controlling the gas supply) and then flows round the oven and out of the vent. The temperature in the middle of the oven corresponds to the thermostat setting, the upper part is about 1 Mark hotter and the bottom is about 1 Mark cooler (temperatures measured with special thermometers). The upper two-thirds of the lighted oven are therefore hotter than the third at the bottom. This enables dishes requiring different temperatures to be cooked at the same time.
By courtesy of British Gas.

Provision is made for the outlet of the products of combustion of the gas by means of an oven flue, and the positions of the burners have a great influence upon the circulation of hot gases in the oven and consequently upon cooking performances. Formerly it was usual to place the flue outlet at the top of the oven, but greater thermal efficiency can be achieved by using a siphon flue with the outlet vent discharging forward over the oven crown plate. This new design reduces the rate of flow of hot gases through the oven and promotes more efficient convection. The heat from the flue gases can be utilised for plate warming where there is a raised plate-rack, and there is no soiling of the wall behind the oven as is the case when the vent is at the back of the oven. The construction of the oven burners is based on the principle of the bunsen flame so as to ensure complete combustion of the gas.

The hottest part of a gas oven is at the top, and there is a temperature fall from the top to the bottom. It is therefore possible to cook foods that require different temperatures at the same time but in different parts of the oven.

However, the fact that the oven temperature varies from shelf to shelf can also be a disadvantage.

Because of the flow of air through a gas oven the outer surface of foods tends to dry and thus they have a crisp outside. If this is not required, the food can be wrapped in metal or plastic film.

The hotplate, or hob, also has burners using the bunsen flame, the commonest type being the drilled ring with spreading flame. It is efficient, it gives good vessel support and is easy to clean. Proper use of the hotplate is important as 75% of the cooking is done on it. The pans used should not be too small in relation to the size of the burner, and the flames should not be allowed to extend beyond the sides of the pan. Finned base kettles save both time and gas.

Thermostatically-controlled burners are now available for the control of the gas burners so that the contents of a pan can be kept simmering. These control the flow of gas by means of a sensory thermostat so that the temperature of the pan contents can be kept constant at a pre-set level.

The grill of the gas cooker is designed to radiate heat on to the surface of food placed a little way below it. The radiating surface—the grill fret—is heated by convection and conduction from the hot

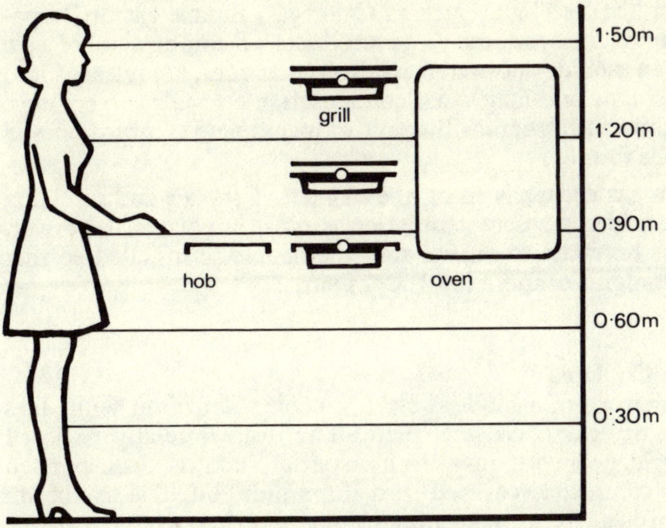

Diagram of an oven showing suggested heights for cooking units.

gases produced by the combustion of gas in a poker-type burner designed so that the flames impinge on the grill fret. The grill pan contains a rack to hold the food during cooking, and, as the best distance between the food and the grill surface is about 50 mm, the rack is made adjustable in height to allow for differences in the thickness of various foods to be grilled.

Gas cookers have the advantages of labour saving. No fuel has to be carried and they do not need stoking. Since there is no heavy dust or smoke, they are easily kept clean. They are extremely flexible in use. Heating by gas to exact times and temperatures is easy because of the immediate response to any adjustment in fuel supply. The gas oven reaches the required temperature, say for roasting, more quickly than the electric or any other type of oven, and is thus faster in cooking and saves time. The gas oven is relatively cheap to hire or purchase and is economical to use since the exact amount of fuel only need be consumed.

The disadvantages of gas cookers are that they cannot be used to heat a water supply nor to heat the kitchen. They cannot be installed in districts without a gas supply although they can be used with "bottled" gas, such as Calor gas, Butane gas or Propagas, supplied in cylinders. The products of combustion of coal gas, carbon dioxide and water, while not harmful, are released into the atmosphere and may cause condensation on walls and ceilings. Poorly adjusted burners will result in incomplete combustion and soot will be formed.

Because a gas cooker is using the oxygen of the air and releasing carbon dioxide adequate ventilation is most important. However, care must be taken to ensure that the cooker is installed so that sudden draughts cannot blow the gas out.

Electric Cookers

The framework of a modern electric cooker is of iron with sides and back of enamelled steel plate. The oven is totally enclosed and well lagged with insulating material such as resin-bonded fibreglass completely covered with aluminium foil. The maximum amount of heat from the heating elements is thus retained for the longest possible time.

For the average household an electric cooker with a three- or four-ring hob is most suitable. Such a cooker would have boiling rings, a grill compartment, an oven and perhaps a separately heated warming drawer. In electric ovens, elements of two types are used, viz., a continuous coil of high-resistance alloy wire which always glows red when a current passes through it, and a tubular sheathed wire element in which the wire is insulated from the sheath by a packing of a mineral oxide and which remains black when a current flows through it. These elements are always protected by guards which help to promote a good air circulation by means of slots and perforations to give the right kind of heat and evenness of browning. The side-guards are designed to hold the oven racks which are "non-tilt" and made of rust-free metal. The guards are vitreous enamelled and removable for easy cleaning. They may also be coated with a "stay–clean" surface.

The heating elements are positioned in the lower halves of the two side walls and bottom or on the side walls only. Bottom heat from the under-flow elements may have some advantages in oven performance but can add to cleaning problems if the oven is used carelessly, spilt food quickly becoming charred on the oven floor and consequently difficult to remove.

In "fan-assisted" ovens a finned heating element of sheathed wire is placed in the centre of the back of the oven. The element does not glow red because of the air current moving over it. A fan in the middle of the element forces the heated air round the oven, producing an even heat distribution throughout the oven.

The boiling rings on electric cookers are of two types which differ both in design and in the method of heat transference. They are the *enclosed* or *solid ring*, which relies on conduction, and the *radiant ring*, which relies mainly on radiation. The enclosed ring consists of one solid plate of an alloy of cast iron containing nickel which is grooved on the underside to house spiral resistance wire embedded in refractory cement. The upper side is machined to give a flat surface, and for efficient use vessels with similar machined bases must be used in conjunction with it to allow the heat from the surface of the boiling ring to pass easily into the vessels.

The radiant ring, which has largely replaced the solid type, consists of a coil of sheathed wire and is similar to that used in the oven, but differs in the maximum temperature reached in use, for while the oven element remains black, that on the boiling ring can become red-hot in use. With this type of boiling ring it is not necessary to use vessels with flat machined bases, for although some of the heat is transferred by conduction where the vessels rest on the element, much more heat comes by radiation from the red-hot element.

The grill of the electric cooker, like that of the gas cooker, is designed to radiate heat on to the surface of food placed a few centimetres beneath it. The *electric grill element* is usually of the sheathed wire type. In most modern cookers it is situated within its own compartment, either at waist-level or at eye-level, but in some of the smaller cookers it can be adapted by using a heat deflector plate to act either as a boiling ring or as a grill. Runners or supports are provided for the grill pan to allow the food to be placed in close proximity to the heat. The grill pans are usually vitreous enamelled and have rounded corners for easy cleaning and reversible racks to give a choice of grilling positions.

All electric ovens are controlled by thermostats similar to those used in gas ovens to give accurate temperature control. They allow the oven to be maintained at any predetermined temperature between 90°C and 280°C. When the selected temperature has been reached the current is switched off automatically and the pilot light in the thermostat control knob goes out. After a short time the light comes on again showing that the mechanism is operating and that the oven temperature is being maintained.

Electric ovens are hottest in the middle and have only a comparatively small range of heat above or below. This is an advantage when baking. A fan set into the back of the oven to circulate the air can provide a uniform heat distribution.

Because electric ovens do not have a flow of air through them they tend to have a higher humidity than gas ovens and meat may not crispen on the outside.

The rings may have either variable or multi-heat control. The infinitely variable heat controls provide an almost unlimited number of settings and can be used to simmer even the smallest quantity of liquid. They operate by opening and closing a knob-action switch in the boiling plate circuit at short definite time intervals. The proportion of time "on" and time "off" is operated by turning the knob in front of the dial.

The auto-time controls fitted to most electric ovens are virtually electric clocks which are connected to a mechanism controlling the oven. They switch the current on and off automatically at predetermined times. They have two main functions: either to switch the current on after a delay at any given time or to switch it off at the expiration of the desired cooking time, or both. Thus food may be placed in a cold oven and auto-cooked from the cold, or the food may be placed in a hot oven and the control set to switch off when the food will be cooked.

The advantages of the electric cooker are that it is easy to use, and labour saving since it requires no fuel-carrying or stoking. It gives a very even heat, produces no smell, dust or smoke, is easily cleaned and is not expensive if used intelligently. An electric oven can be placed practically anywhere in the kitchen—there is no restriction in the siting of the oven since the fixing of a flue or the problem of draughts do not arise. There are, of course, no flue gases from an electric oven.

Its disadvantages are that it does not heat the water supply, cannot be used to warm the kitchen, takes some time to reach the desired temperature and can only be used in districts where there is an electricity supply.

Electronic (Micro-Wave) Cookers

Electronic ovens are not yet widely available in this country, though some are in use in restaurants, but they have been used in the U.S.A. for some years. These ovens utilise the energy in the high-frequency radio wave band to cook the food. Micro-waves generated by a magnetron are beamed on to the food, penetrate it to a depth of about 75 mm and produce heat internally. The heating times required are very short and there is a complete absence of heat in the oven. Electronically cooked food has a somewhat different appearance from that cooked in a conventional oven. In the latter, the outside surfaces of the food reach the highest temperature and usually turn brown. In the electronic oven, the waves penetrate towards the centre of the food and are absorbed evenly throughout, but the outside surfaces do not brown. Containers made of china, glass and some plastics transmit these micro-waves and can be used in the electronic oven. Metal containers cannot be used because metals reflect these rays.

REFRIGERATORS

Larders are seldom efficient in storing and preserving perishable foods, and a refrigerator for these purposes is desirable. A refrigerator provides storage space at a temperature lower than its surroundings in which perishable foods can be kept in first-class condition for a reasonable period of time independent of external conditions. Wastage of food is thus reduced, the risk of food contamination and food poisoning very largely eliminated, and the buying and storing of food simplified. In addition, packets of quick-frozen foods can be stored for varying periods, ice is available for iced drinks, bottled drinks can be chilled, ice-cream can be made and a whole range of new cold dishes can be prepared. A much greater variety in the menu is possible. Unfortunately, not everyone in this country is able to afford a refrigerator, but the day will come when every working kitchen will be fitted with this essential piece of equipment.

Those able to afford a refrigerator should make sure that it is big enough for their needs and should look after it carefully by keeping the door shut and "defrosting" it regularly. A refrigerator of ample size—30 litres of storage space for each member of the

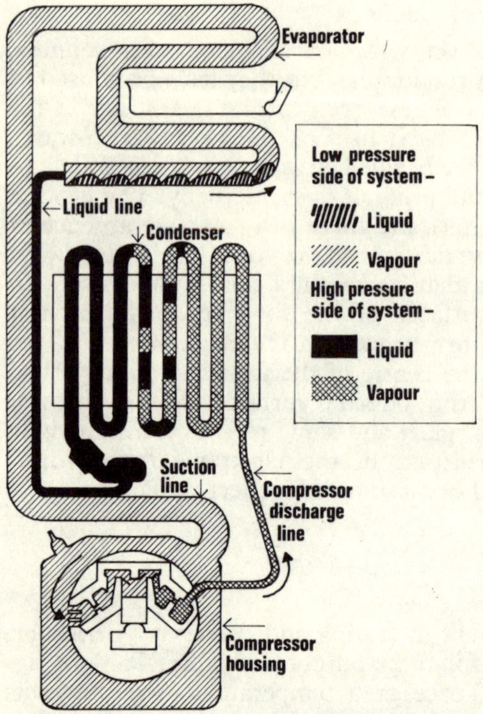

The working of an electric refrigerator. By courtesy of the Food Freezer and Refrigerator Council.

household—a smaller cupboard on the wall and a vegetable cupboard under a counter top make a larder unnecessary.

The micro-organisms which cause decay in foods, i.e., yeasts, moulds and bacteria, grow fastest at temperatures between 27°C, and 33°C. At temperatures between 5°C and 12°C growth of these organisms is slowed down but not completely stopped. Thus food cannot be kept wholesome for more than a day or two, the time varying with the type of food. In the domestic refrigerator the controls are kept not at freezing point (0°C), but at a higher temperature, the normal range being between 5°C and 12°C. This temperature is suitable for storing such things as milk, meat, fish and vegetables, but the period during which they can be preserved at such temperatures is generally limited to a few days.

There is one part of the refrigerator, however, where a temperature below freezing is maintained, and this is within the ice box. The actual temperature of the ice box will depend on the type of refrigerator. Modern refrigerators are now given star ratings which guarantee the maximum temperature of the ice box.

A one-star rating indicates that the maximum temperature will be −6°C. This is sufficient to store frozen foods for 1 week.

A two-star rating indicates that the maximum temperature will be −12°C. This is sufficient to store frozen foods for 1 month.

A three-star rating indicates that the maximum temperature will be −18°C. This is sufficient to store frozen foods for three months.

None of these "star-marked" compartments should be used to actually freeze the food.

Many modern refrigerators have a chiller drawer immediately below the ice box where fish, meat, bacon and cooked meats can be stored. The vegetable drawer, often glass-covered at the base of a refrigerator, is suitable for storage of vegetables and fruit, the glass actually reduces the flow of air and there is less tendency for the vegetables to dry up.

Food freezers are capable of freezing a specified weight of fresh or cooked food from +25°C to −18°C in 24 hours, as well as storing already-frozen food. These freezers are marked with the three-star marking and a larger star in a different colour. The weight of food that can be frozen daily must be specified by the manufacturer and should not be exceeded, or the quality of the food will be inferior.

Apart from the types of freezer mentioned below, a combination refrigerator/freezer is available, either housed in one cabinet but with two doors, or consisting of two completely separate units, usually fitted one above the other.

A capacity of 75 litres per person is advisable.

Food freezers may be of two types. A: the chest type where the lid of the chest is hinged at the top. The food is stored in baskets. This type of freezer allows awkward-sized food to be

s

stored and there is less heat loss when the lid is opened than with the upright type of freezer. The chest freezer will probably require defrosting once a year. The disadvantages are the amount of floor space it occupies and the fact that the food is stored on top of itself.

B: the upright, front-opening type of freezer is more like the conventional refrigerator with a side-hinged door, and shelves. Food is more accessible, but opening the door causes a heat exchange and more frequent defrosting is necessary with this type of freezer.

Electric and gas refrigerators are made but both work upon the same basic principles and only differ in details. A liquid boils when its vapour pressure is equal to that of the surrounding atmosphere. Thus, water boils when it is heated to 100°C because at that temperature its vapour pressure becomes equal to that of the atmosphere. Alternatively, a liquid may be made to boil by reducing the external pressure until it is equal to the vapour pressure of the liquid. In order to evaporate at this reduced pressure the liquid absorbs heat from its surroundings. In this way intense cold can be produced by the rapid evaporation of a liquid under reduced pressure. This is precisely what takes place in a refrigerator.

Refrigerators are of two types; the compression type and the absorption type. Those worked by electricity are usually compression refrigerators and those worked by gas, always absorption.

The compression refrigerator has four main parts: the food-storage chamber, the compressor, the condenser, and the evaporator or "frozen food compartment". These components are usually assembled in one cabinet with the food-storage chamber surrounded by insulating material, such as granulated cork, expanded plastic, or slag wool, to prevent heat passing through from the outside. Some chemical substance which is easily liquefied by pressure, e.g., Freon–12 or Arcton–6, or dichloro-difluoromethane, is used as the refrigerant.

The continuous cycle of operations, which is controlled by a thermostat, is briefly as follows. The compressor, which is driven by a small electric motor, exerts pressure upon the gaseous refrigerant which at the same time is cooled in the condenser by the air outside the refrigerator. The refrigerant is thus liquefied

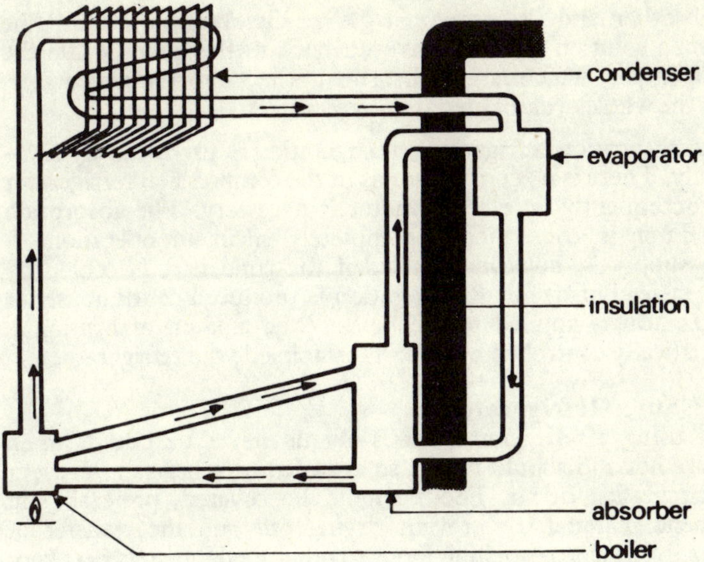

The working of a gas refrigerator. By courtesy of British Gas.

and in this form passes in small amounts to the evaporator where it expands and evaporates. In its evaporation it absorbs heat from the food-storage chamber which is thus cooled. The gaseous refrigerant is then drawn into the compressor again and reliquefied. This cycle of operations is continuous and heat is abstracted from the storage chamber at each cycle. The controlling thermostat is in the form of bellows which contain a gas. The expansion and contraction of this gas with rise and fall in temperature switches the electric motor on or off when suitable minimum and maximum temperatures are reached.

The absorption refrigerator has a solution of ammonia gas in water as its refrigerant. The ammonia gas is liberated from its solution in water by a small gas flame, electric element, oil burner or even a "bottled" gas burner, under the boiler. The ammonia gas then passes to the condenser where it is liquefied by means of water or air circulating round it. The liquefied ammonia is led into the evaporator with some hydrogen where it expands and changes to ammonia gas with the absorption of heat from the food-storage chamber which is thus cooled. The gases produced are then led to the absorber and the ammonia gas re-dissolved in water. The ammonia solution is then conveyed back to the boiler while the hydrogen gas, which is not absorbed, is led into the evaporator. Thus the whole cycle of operations is completed.

In the absorption refrigerator, refrigeration is produced by heating only. There is no compressor as in the compression refrigerator and consequently no electric motor is necessary. The absorption refrigerator is consequently completely silent in operation. A water supply is, however, needed if the condenser is cooled by water instead of by air. Refrigeration is produced continuously as long as heat is applied to the boiler. The amount of heating is automatically controlled by a thermostat inside the refrigerator.

The use of a Refrigerator

When using a refrigerator, foods should never be put in when they are hot and should not be so crowded together as to prevent free circulation of air. Foods should be covered, preferably in polythene material, to prevent drying out and the transfer of odours from strong-smelling foods to other foods. Fish is best kept in the freezer tray beneath the freezing compartment. Ice-cream and quick-frozen foods should be placed in the freezing compartment. The door of the refrigerator should be kept tightly closed and only opened when necessary. Finally, the refrigerator should always be kept clean, inside and out, and defrosted, i.e., excessive ice removed from the evaporator or "freezer," at regular intervals.

Defrosting

There are three possible methods of defrosting:

1. Manual defrosting
2. Semi-automatic defrosting
3. Fully-automatic defrosting.

1. Manual defrosting is done by turning the control dial to "off" or "defrost." The food is then removed and as the ice melts the water will be collected in the drip tray. A dish of hot water in the freezing compartment will hasten the melting of the ice. When all the ice has melted the refrigerator should be wiped out and the dial reset for the desired degree of refrigeration.

2. Semi-automatic defrosting is done by pressing a defrost button. This turns the refrigeration unit off and when the ice has melted

the refrigerator will switch itself on again. Sometimes a heater is present to speed up the rate of defrosting. The manufacturer will give instruction about the removal of food.

3. Automatic defrosting. This takes place automatically at frequent intervals so that there is no build-up of ice and there is no need to remove the food.

20 Small Equipment

KETTLES

For the average small household a $1\frac{1}{2}$–litre kettle is the most convenient size, and a good quality aluminium kettle is most suitable. Time and fuel will be saved if the kettle has a finned base. Tin kettles do not last long and copper kettles take time to polish. For electric cookers of the hotplate type an immersion-heated electric kettle is needed to save fuel. With solid-fuel cookers, close contact with hotplate is essential for quick boiling. A heavy aluminium kettle with a machined bottom or ground base is most suitable.

All kettles should have spouts which pour cleanly without dripping. The handle should be insulated and firmly riveted. It should be so shaped as to allow it to be grasped without the hand getting into the direct line of steam when the lid is off for refilling. The lid should fit well and have a strong edge to withstand hard wear. The knob should be insulated and securely fixed. A small vent in the lid to allow steam to escape prevents the lid from rattling and the water from bubbling over when the kettle boils.

SAUCEPANS

For the average small household the essential minimum is three lidded saucepans of different sizes and a "milk" saucepan with a lip. The first consideration in purchasing saucepans, apart from cost, is the material of which they are made. The two commonest materials are aluminium and enamel, but stainless steel, copper, brass, glass, Monel metal, nickel, tinned steel and cast iron are also available. Ideally, the material used for saucepans should be durable; hard enough to resist scratching, pitting, abrasives and knocks; strong enough to retain its shape under strain; resistant to moisture, acids and alkalis; non-poisonous; easy to clean and a good conductor of heat. Of whatever material it is made, a thin pan will heat up more quickly and be lighter to handle while thicker metal will be more resistant to dents and burnt spots.

First quality aluminium pans, either cast or wrought, are very durable, but light gauge wrought or poor quality cast aluminium are much less satisfactory. Aluminium is not very hard and its resistance to scratching, pitting, abrasives and knocks is not very high. Nor is it particularly easy to clean, and hard rubbing with fine steel wool and soap is frequently necessary. The film of oxide on the surface of aluminium is not normally attacked by moisture, but mild alkalis and organic acids will dissolve it. The film will reform immediately afterwards, but obviously this process cannot go on indefinitely. A black stain often remains after boiling tap water in an aluminium pan, probably because of the presence of small amounts of iron in the water. This stain can be removed by mild abrasives or by solution in boiling water containing a little vinegar. Finally, aluminium is non-poisonous, light in weight and a good conductor of heat.

Enamel ware is reasonably hard wearing provided good quality products are purchased. Enamel is hard and resistant to scratching and pitting, but the constant use of abrasives spoils the original shining surface. Because of its glass-like nature, the enamel coating will chip and crack if dropped, banged or overheated. Since enamel ware is made of cast iron or sheet steel it is, of course, very strong. When new, the smooth, shiny surface is easy to clean but becomes more difficult as the surface becomes dull and roughened and still more difficult when it is chipped. An undamaged enamelled surface is completely resistant to moisture, but once the surface is broken and the iron underneath exposed rusting is difficult to prevent. Enamel is not as good a conductor as aluminium and is consequently not as good for heating milk or making sauces which have a tendency to scorch. A black base and white sides are best; the former absorbs the heat readily and the latter reduces heat loss to a minimum.

Stainless steel pans are very expensive but have a very long life and all the desirable qualities previously enumerated except that of high thermal conductivity, and such a pan would scorch milk or sauces as readily as an enamel pan. This disadvantage can be overcome by cladding the bottom outside surface with another metal which is a good conductor of heat, e.g., brass, copper or aluminium. The main advantage of copper and brass as materials for pans is their high thermal conductivity which makes such pans very suitable for jam-making and sauce-making, while scorching is highly unlikely. Copper is hard-wearing, strong and reasonably hard but corrodes readily to form a poisonous film. Constant cleaning is thus necessary for the sake of safety as well as of appearance. This disadvantage can be overcome by lining the inside of the pan with a non-corrosive metal such as tin or nickel. Brass is comparable to copper except that it is harder, more resistant to corrosion and not quite as good a conductor of heat. Copper and brass are expensive and may be heavy.

"Non-stick" pans

Silicone-lined pans avoid sticking or burning of the food. This makes them easy to clean. They should not be touched with abrasives, and only wooden implements should be used for stirring in them.

A coating of polytetrafluorethylene (PTFE) can also be used. If (as in the Teflon process) prior to the use of this coating the metal is coated with a layer of particles producing a ridged surface, a more scratch-resistant surface will be produced than if the surface was quite flat. This means that metal implements can be used with the pans (e.g. omelettes are stirred with a fork in the traditional way). Harsh scourers and abrasive powders should not, however, be used in cleaning. Hot water and detergent, followed by rinsing, are all that is necessary.

Both the base coat and the PTFE coating have to be baked on at a high temperature, and so this coating can only be put on to metal or glass. However, in actual cooking, very high temperatures should be avoided. Overheating sometimes produces stains on the pans, and these can be lightened by boiling in the pan a mixture of 2 tablespoons baking powder, ½ cup liquid household bleach and 1 cup of water, for about 5–10 minutes. This treatment should be followed by thorough washing, rinsing and drying, and a little salad oil may be wiped over the pan before it is next used.

Next to the material of the pan, the design is an important consideration. Round pans are the most usual since they are most suitable if the contents have to be stirred and they are the easiest shape to clean. Square pans are convenient for use on rectangular electric boiling plates since two such pans can be placed closely side by side. The junction of the sides and base of the pan should

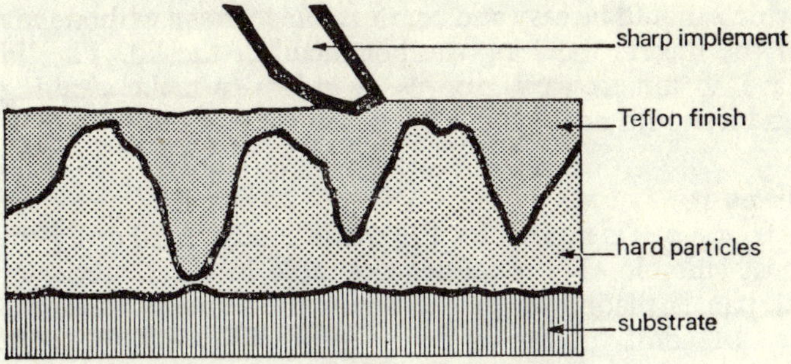

Enlarged cross-section of a scratch-resistant Teflon coating.
The hard particles on the substrate protect the coating against the sharp edges of metal utensils.
By courtesy of Dupont de Nemours International S.A.

be curved for easier cleaning and stirring, and not a sharp corner at right angles as is often the case. For electric or solid-fuel hotplates it is essential that the saucepans should be absolutely flat-based so as to make complete contact with the hotplate.

All handles should be insulated so that they can be safely grasped with the bare hand when in use. Some metal handles are insulated by covering them with plastic and some are made in the form of a hollow tube sealed at the end. Other handles are made of wood because it is a poor conductor of heat. Such handles, however, may become charred if used carelessly on a gas cooker and will deteriorate if left in water for long periods. Of whatever material it is made, the handle should be comfortable to grip and not too long for convenience. The weight of the handle relative to that of the empty pan should not be such as to spoil the balance of the pan, i.e., the pan should not topple when empty.

The method of fixing the handle to the pan is an important factor because it is at this point that the greatest strain is felt, and many handles work loose after a time. Welding is the best method for fixing iron and steel but is difficult with aluminium, for which rivets are usually used which eventually work loose. Some cast aluminium pans have a handle boss cast with the pan and a metal handle covered with plastic riveted to this boss, thus avoiding rivets on the inside surface of the pan.

The lids should be strong and well-fitting with insulated knobs or handles which should be easy and comfortable to grasp without any danger of the fingers touching the hot metal of the lid. The lid should have no unnecessary grooves or ridges to make cleaning difficult and it should not be liable to stick in the pan.

Frying pans

Only one frying pan is needed for the small family. A 20 or 24 cm pan is most suitable. The qualities desirable in the material of which the pan is made are, in the main, the same as those for saucepans. In addition, the material must withstand the high temperatures used for frying, 180°–200° C, without buckling and becoming distorted. It is thus even more important than with saucepans that the frying pan should be of heavy gauge material so as not to buckle. Thin pans easily buckle and fry unevenly with the result that in some spots the food is burnt and in others uncooked. Because of the high temperature involved, the handle should be well insulated, and sealed as well as firmly riveted. The whole pan should be well balanced and the corners at the base, as with saucepans, should be curved to facilitate cleaning.

For deep fat frying, the pan should be deep but not too wide and should be fitted with a strainer.

STEAMERS

Steamers can be purchased which fit several sizes of saucepans, but with large saucepans they are liable to sink so far in as to leave little room for cooking anything underneath. With tiered steamers it is possible to cook a whole dinner on one burner or hotplate. Steamer handles and the knob on the lid should be insulated.

PRESSURE COOKERS

There are two main types of pressure cookers on the market. The larger and more robust type, e.g., Easiwork, is fitted with clock pressure and temperature gauge, safety valve and pressure regulator or "whistle." Any type of cooking, whether it be steaming, roasting, baking or deep fat frying can be quickly carried out in these cookers, as well as the making of preserves and the bottling of fruits and vegetables. These cookers can be adjusted to cook at a range of pressures by means of the whistle pressure regulator which must always be in perfect working order.

The smaller, cheaper and simpler type, such as the Presto, consists of a deep aluminium saucepan with a lid that locks on tightly and is fitted with a safety valve to release excess pressure. With this type of pressure cooker there is a choice of three pressures.

CASSEROLES

At least two casseroles with lids are advisable. Casseroles hold the heat well and can be used on the table and so save dishing and washing up. They may be made of earthenware, glass or metal with various finishes. The best types are those with a lid that can be used as a separate dish when required. Casseroles made of special heat-resisting glasses, such as Pyrex and Phoenix, are particularly suitable. In addition to the silicates of which ordinary glass is composed, they contain borates which enable them to withstand very high temperatures without softening. Their coefficient of expansion is lower than that of ordinary glass. Consequently they can be quickly cooled without danger of cracking.

Pyrosil ware is made of glass with an exceptionally high heat conductivity. It can be used on a hotplate or on the naked gas flame and can be immediately plunged into cold water.

Some casseroles are made with detachable handles so that they can be used as saucepans.

ROASTING TINS, BAKING TINS, CAKE TINS

One roasting tin, one baking tray, one cake tin (150 mm), two sandwich tins (200 mm), two bun tins to hold twelve buns each and one deep plate will probably meet average requirements. All should be of good heavy quality so as not to buckle or cause food to burn. Cakes baked in thin tins will rise and brown unevenly. Tins with rolled edges do not cut the hands, are stronger and keep their shape better than those with unrolled edges. In addition, liquids and grease are prevented from falling into the oven. The tins may be made of non-rusting tin-plate or aluminium. Roasting tins and baking trays should fit comfortably into the oven and leave at least 50 mm all round to allow free circulation of hot air.

Non-stick and scratch-resistant-non-stick finishes are available on roasting, baking and cake tins but light greasing is still advisable.

CUTTING AND ALLIED TOOLS

The qualities necessary in knife blades are that they should hold a good edge, resist corrosion and staining, withstand chipping and breaking and, except for chopping knives, be flexible. The choice of materials is restricted to carbon steel and stainless steel, the latter being much the more common. Carbon steel blades will take and hold a good cutting edge much better than stainless steel but readily stain and corrode and require constant care and cleaning with bathbrick. Stainless steel blades are as sharp as carbon steel when new but cannot be as easily re-sharpened on a steel or carborundum; they require grinding. To overcome this serious defect many stainless steel blades are now hollow ground or fluted or have the Granton edge. This gives a very satisfactory cutting edge but the metal is so thin as to make it liable to chip unless treated carefully. Stainless steel does not, of course, stain or corrode in use.

The handle of the knife may be of hardwood, rosewood, bone or plastic. Whatever material is used should be impervious to water and should not chip or break easily. It should feel comfortable in the hand and, in the case of a chopping knife, should be so shaped that the fingers will not strike the table when it is used for chopping. The metal continuation of the blade, the tang, can be fixed into the handle with either glue or rivets. The latter type is preferable for kitchen use as it is stronger; glue is apt to soften when the knife is left soaking in hot water.

A sharp-pointed vegetable knife and a good medium-sized cook's knife for chopping are essential. Other knives, e.g., a saw knife for slicing tomatoes and vegetables and a saw-edged breadknife, are also needed. A broad-bladed palette knife with rounded end, which is flexible enough to bend to the shape of a mixing bowl for scraping out and afterwards return to its original shape, is desirable. So also is a stout pair of easily handled scissors.

A knife sharpener of the hard steel disc type can be used for both carbon steel and stainless steel blades and does not mark or scratch the blade. The familiar "steel" can be used for carbon steel knives and so can carborundum sharpeners. Knives should never be sharpened on the kitchen step nor should they be used for purposes for which they were never intended. Knives are neither screwdrivers nor tin-openers! Remember too that the knife edge will remain sharp much longer if a wooden board is used as the cutting surface rather than the much harder surfaces of steel, Formica or earthenware.

Many people prefer a potato peeler to a knife. It is quicker and more economical in use. A can opener of the "handle into jaws" or rotary type and a few forks are other essential small items of kitchen equipment. A two-pronged fork is useful for dishing and so on.

SPOONS

The following metal spoons will be needed: a tablespoon, dessert spoon, teaspoon, cook's perforated spoon and a soup ladle. The last two should have handles of wood or other insulating material. All spoons should be simple in design, well-shaped, comfortable to hold and robust without being clumsy. A set of measuring spoons is of great assistance in cooking. (See page 261.)

Two or three wooden spoons of varying sizes are needed for stirring sauces, batters, jam and so on. They should be of hard, close-grained wood so as not to splinter or lose their smooth finish. Their shape should be such as to make contact with the bottom and corners of pans possible. Rounded wooden spoons are better than oval but the best spoons are level at the bottom.

WHISKS

Whisks may be of the hand type or rotary type. The hand type is preferable for whisking small quantities and the rotary type for larger quantities of eggs.

ELECTRIC MIXERS

The aim of an electric mixer is to do mechanically many of the basic physical activities of cooking. The simplest type of mixer is a hand-held electric whisk. Some of the light mixing machines have a variety of beaters for different types of mixing, some are provided with a stand.

The heavier and more powerful mixers cannot be hand-held, are capable of beating heavier mixtures and usually have a variety of attachments that can be used for blending, shredding etc. Some of these machines can be installed into a working surface or within a drawer.

PASTRY BOARDS AND ROLLING PINS

A pastry board is unnecessary if the table or counter has a hardwood, aluminium or enamelled or laminated plastic top. A piece of American cloth will serve the same purpose. If a pastry board is used it may be of wood or pottery. Wooden boards should be made of evenly grained hard wood, free from knots. Pottery and marble boards give a cool surface which is easy to keep perfectly clean.

Whether made of hardwood, glass, china, plastic or aluminium, the rolling pin should be straight, smooth and fairly heavy. If the handles are loose it is easier to roll lightly. "Non-stick" rolling pins are beginning to come into use.

The pastry board should not be used as a chopping board. A separate hardwood board should be used for this.

A pastry brush is useful and should have its bristles firmly secured to the handle since it has to stand up to cleaning in very hot water.

STRAINERS, SIEVES AND COLANDERS

It is best to have a coffee strainer, a pointed strainer and a round strainer. They should have a hook on the rim opposite the handle to fit over the vessel into which the liquid is being strained. The wire mesh should be strong and should fit perfectly into the rim.

Sieves are made of wire or plastic and have meshes of various sizes. The wire should be lightly and firmly fixed into the frame. Wooden frames are more durable than all-metal ones.

Colanders may be of enamelled iron, aluminium or plastic and can be purchased with or without handles. The usual size has a diameter of 250 mm. The holes should be smoothly finished, the surface rustless and the colander should stand firmly on its base.

GRATERS

Two-way graters with the teeth set in alternate rows, one row facing downwards and the next upwards, are most suitable for grating raw vegetables, cheese and bread crumbs, since they give continuous grating with both upward and downward movements of the hand. Wire mesh graters serve the same purpose and have the advantage of not grating the fingers. Graters of both types should be so shaped as either to stand up in a bowl or to hook on to the bowl without slipping.

Graters may be coarse, medium or fine. Coarse graters are used for suet and vegetables, medium for bread crumbs and fine for nutmegs. The three types can be combined in round or three screen graters. All graters should be rustless and easy to clean. If it can be afforded, a rotary mill is excellent for nuts and cheese.

SCALES AND MEASURING CUPS AND SPOONS

Good kitchen scales are a necessity if reliable results are to be obtained. The two main types are the beam type with separate weights and the spring balance type which shows the weight on a dial. The beam type is more accurate and lasts longer. Whichever type is chosen it should be sufficiently sensitive to weigh small amounts accurately. The 2·5 kg size will be big enough for the small family. The weights of the beam scale should be Government-stamped. The pan may be plain or enamelled metal or plastic. It should rest firmly and evenly on the scales. Scoop-shaped pans make for easier pouring than round ones.

Measuring cups and spoons are obtainable for use with recipes where cupfuls and spoonfuls are given instead of grammes and litres. The cups may be half litre with smaller quantities clearly marked or a nest of cups, one for each quantity. Lipped cups for liquids and unlipped cups for dry goods can be purchased. The measuring spoons are circular to make them more accurate. Recipes are now often written with British Standard measuring cups and spoons in mind.

BOWLS, BASINS AND JUGS

Mixing bowls should be of a good size, say 300 mm, as beating and mixing are more easily done in a large bowl than a small one. The sides should be slightly curved to prevent food from being scattered during beating.

Pudding basins should have well-moulded rims to allow paper or cloth to be tied to them easily and securely.

Jugs should have wide level bases so that they are not easily knocked over and wide mouths so that they can easily be cleaned. The spouts should enable pouring to be done without dripping. The handles should be easy to grasp and without ornamentation which collects dirt and makes cleaning difficult.

The glaze of all earthenware should be even, hard and leadless.

STORAGE JARS, TINS AND BINS

Glass storage jars with rustless screw-top lids are excellent for storing cereals, pulses and other dry food. It is easy to see how the foods are keeping and when they need replenishing. Pottery jars are good and aluminium containers are light and rustless. Plastic containers are becoming increasingly popular. Tea, coffee and spices should be stored in airtight containers to avoid loss of aroma and flavour. Baking powder should be kept dry in a sealed tin. Salt should preferably be stored in a glass container. Enamelled bins and tins are necessary for flour, bread, cakes, biscuits and so on.

KITCHEN CLOTHS, PAPER, POLYTHENE AND FOIL

Tea towels are best made of linen or a mixture of linen and cotton. They wear longer and absorb moisture more easily than cotton. Dishcloths are woven from strong coarse cotton which does not easily fluff and clog the drain. An oven cloth of canvas, hessian or other strong material should always be kept handy. Facilities for drying kitchen cloths are a necessity and special rails can be purchased for the purpose. A sink shelf for the smaller sink accessories is a handy piece of equipment.

Paper has many uses in the kitchen. Greaseproof paper has obvious uses in lining cake tins, wrapping foods and as a protection against burning in baking. Small waxed circles are used to protect jams and marmalades from air, moisture and moulds. Double-waxed opaque papers in sheet form are available for wrapping food and sandwiches. Kitchen paper rolls are suitable for cleaning, draining or drying and covering kitchen utensils and many kinds of food. Once used the pieces of paper are simply thrown away. Non-woven cloths are stronger and washable, but can harbour germs and should not be re-used too often.

Polythene in sheet or bag form is being increasingly used in the kitchen as a wrapping material for food, particularly in conjunction with the refrigerator. Aluminium foil is widely used for wrapping foods, especially in the cooking of joints and poultry.

Plastic film is available for wrapping food to be stored in the refrigerator. It can also be used to cover joints of meat etc., which are to be roasted in the oven as it withstands heat. As the film is transparent it allows the cook to see how the food is progressing.

VEGETABLE RACKS

A vegetable rack near the sink where the vegetables are to be washed is a great convenience. All vegetables remain fresh longer if they are kept cool. Root vegetables are best stored in a rack which allows cold air to circulate freely round them. The shelves may be perforated or of strong wire mesh. The vegetable rack should be simply constructed of rustless material and easily cleaned. Salad greens, provided they are dry, are best kept in a cool airtight container, e.g., pan with a lid. Greens of the cabbage type need air in storing.

GARBAGE BINS

Kitchen refuse may be organic or inorganic. Such organic refuse as peelings, scrapings from plates, tealeaves, etc., should not be carelessly thrown into a food bin where it will speedily decay, causing unpleasant smells and attracting flies. Suitable food waste may be given to animals or poultry and some will be suitable for garden compost. Otherwise, all organic refuse should be burned. If this is not possible, it should be dried and wrapped tightly in newspaper before it is put into the bin. Food bins should be of rustless metal or plastic, have tight-fitting lids to keep out flies and should be easy to clean. They should be frequently cleaned and dried. Paper or polythene lining bags that can be sealed before being put in the dustbin can be used inside the food bins. Paper bags impregnated with plastic are stronger, or plastic bags can be used on their own clipped on to a plastic or metal lid.

Electric food waste disposers which fit into the sink rely on a flow of water to wash down finely shredded waste. Basically they are of two types, one in which the refuse is put into the machine before it is switched on, whereas the other type is switched on and then fed with refuse. The refuse is shredded by rotating steel blades. All food waste can be disposed of in this way but not metal, glass, string or plastic which will damage or clog the blades. Some machines have a reverse gear to help in case the blades become jammed, some have extra sound insulation.

Inorganic refuse such as ashes, soot, broken crockery and empty tins should be placed in the dustbin. This should be of galvanised iron, rubber or plastic, round in shape, with handles for carrying, and a rounded base raised from the floor by a metal rim. The

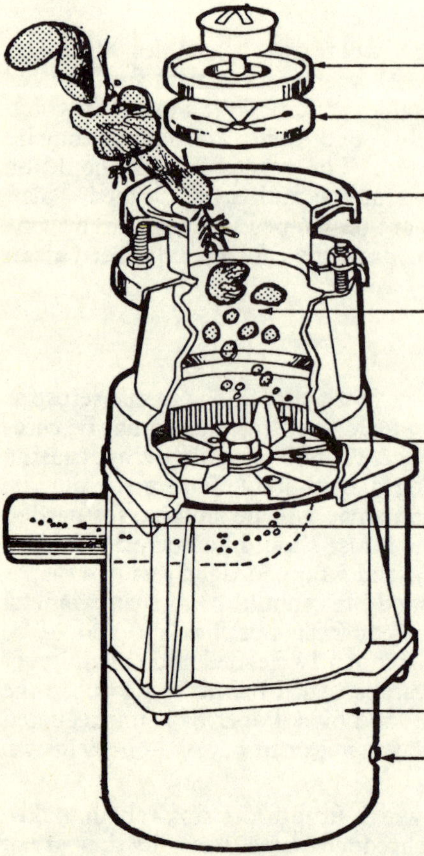

Cross-section of the "Kenwood Waste-away" disposer.
By courtesy of Kenwood Manufacturing (Woking) Limited.

rubber and plastic bins are lighter and less noisy than metal ones and have the advantage that if dented by rough usage they easily regain their shape, so that the rim remains circular and the fit of the lid is not impaired. Often they have an arrangement of slots and projections for bolting the lids on to the rims. Hot ashes should not be put directly into such bins but left in a metal receptacle until cool.

The dustbin should be frequently and regularly emptied and placed conveniently near the house but not close to the larder or open windows. After emptying, the dustbin should be disinfected.

Disposable plastic and also paper sacks of considerable toughness and wet-strength fixed on special holders fitted with a lid are also available for refuse collections and are provided by some local authorities.

BRUSHES

Brushes specifically for kitchen work will include a short-bristled saucepan brush with a straight handle, a bottle brush and a small stiff brush, about 100 mm long, for scrubbing vegetables.

METERS

If gas or electricity is installed, a meter will also be fitted. This should be where it can easily be cleaned and the dial seen.

Most electricity meters have a number of dials similar to the meter illustrated below. When reading a meter, write down the readings of the dials from left to right, ignoring the one reading 1/10ths units. When a pointer is between two figures write down the smaller one. (If the pointer is between 9 and 0 write down 9.) When a pointer is almost on a figure write down one less except when the hand on the next dial has just passed 0. Read the meter weekly and by subtracting last week's reading from this week's you can find

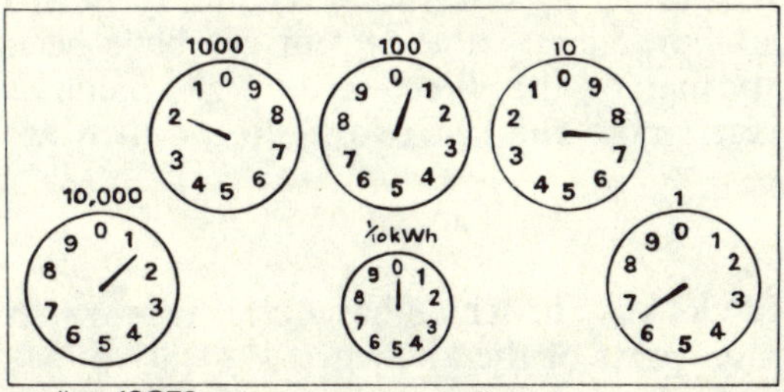

Reading of an electricity meter.

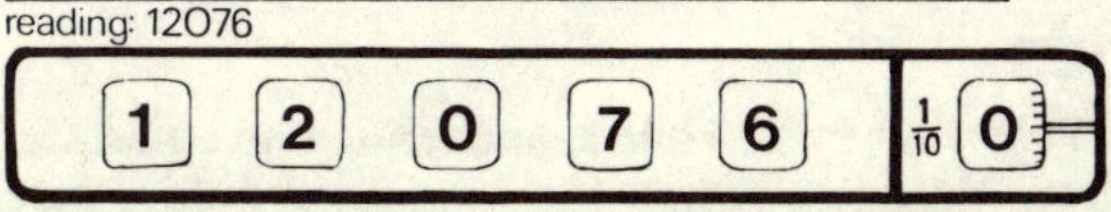

Direct-reading meter reproduced from a Department of Trade and Industry booklet by permission of the Controller of Her Majesty's Stationery Office.

out how many units have been used. Some meters have no dials and are called direct-reading meters. There is no difficulty in reading these, just ignore the number in the last window (labelled 1/10).

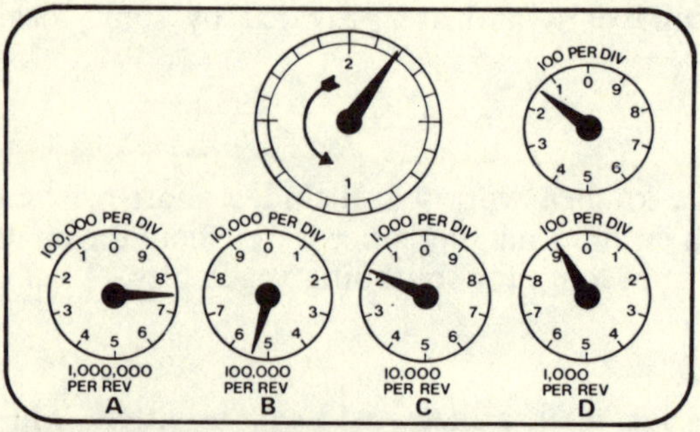

Reading of a gas meter.
By courtesy of British Gas

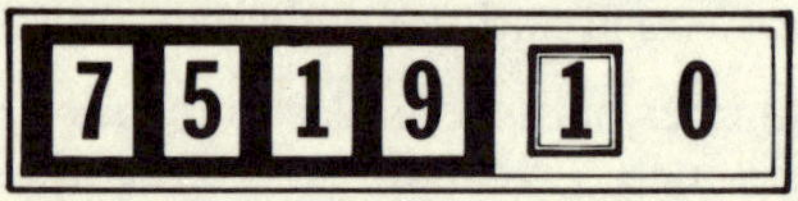

Reading 7519, ie: 751900 cubic feet

A gas meter, like most electricity meters, also has a row of dials, as shown in the illustration above. When reading a meter, only read the four dials at the bottom (the top two dials usually have red hands). Write down the readings of the dials from left to right as with an electricity meter. Since the readings will be in hundreds of cubic feet your total figure must be multiplied by 100, i.e., 00 must be added to it. By subtracting last week's reading from this week's you can find out how many cubic feet of gas have been used. As with electricity meters, the direct-reading gas meter is much easier to read, just ignore the last two figures, which are usually red.

CLOCK

The best type of kitchen clock is one which has a clear face which can easily be seen from all parts of the kitchen.

MISCELLANEOUS

A tin opener, mincer, corkscrew and bottle opener, lemon squeezer, fish slice, funnel, flour dredger, pastry cutters, jelly moulds, wire cake rack, grapefruit knife, sugar-boiler's thermometer, icing tubes and bags are other small items which will find a place in a completely equipped kitchen.

PART FIVE

21 The Planning of Meals

We must begin this chapter by a recapitulation of the main facts given in Chapter 1. We saw there that an adequate diet should provide (i) the necessary kcals to supply the required energy, (ii) proteins and minerals for building and repair, and (iii) vitamins and minerals to supply protective materials. We saw, too, that the body derives its energy mainly from fats and carbohydrates such as butter, margarine, suet, lard, dripping, cereals, pulses, sugar, treacle, jam, syrup, cheese, bacon and ham; its body-building materials from milk, eggs, meat, fish and cheese supplemented by cereals, pulses and nuts; and its protective materials from the minerals and vitamins of milk, cream, butter, eggs, cheese, summer fruits, foreign citrus fruits, vegetables, particularly salad vegetables, fat fish and liver.

It was also pointed out that it was unnecessary for the housewife to calculate the number of kilocalories, the amounts of protein, this particular vitamin, or that particular mineral she was supplying in the daily diet of her family. We suggested that a diet made up of the following foods would provide all the necessary nutrients:

(1) *Milk*. At least ½ litre daily and more for children and expectant and nursing mothers.

(2) *Eggs, cheese and pulses*. At least three or four times per week.

(3) *Meat, fish or poultry*. Once daily.

(4) *Fruit*. Orange, grapefruit or tomato at least once daily.

(5) *Vegetables*. Two kinds daily in addition to potatoes and including one salad or green vegetable.

(6) *Fat*. Butter or vitaminised margarine.

(7) *Cereals*. Wheatflour is the most valuable.

(8) *Water*. About 1¼ litres of fluids daily, some in the form of water, the rest as beverages.

Then eat any other foods you like in order to satisfy your appetite. The more varied the diet the less likely it is to be deficient in any one nutrient.

The housewife's problem is to arrange these foods in the form of meals in such a way as not only to provide the necessary kilocalories, protein, minerals, vitamins, roughage and water, but to do so in such a way as to make them attractive, palatable, satisfying, digestible and economical.

The following rules may be helpful in planning the menu:

(1) The whole day, or better still, the whole week, should be regarded as the unit rather than each individual meal. Any deficiencies in one meal can be made up in the others.

(2) The same foods should not be served more than once in the same day without varying the form in which they are served. This does not apply to such staple foods as milk, bread, butter and margarine.

(3) The same food should not be served twice in the same meal even in different form.

(4) The colour, form and texture of different courses should be varied as much as possible to avoid monotony. A soft food should be alternated with a crisp food that needs chewing; a bland food with a highly seasoned one; cooked food with raw food and so on.

(5) No meal should contain too great a concentration of any one type of nutrient, i.e., no meal should be predominantly protein or fat or carbohydrate in character. As previously pointed out, it is particularly important that both protein and fat should be accompanied by carbohydrate at the same meal.

(6) Serve the animal proteins—milk, eggs, meat, cheese and fish—in small quantities at each meal rather than concentrate them in one meal. In this way the body makes better use of their building material particularly if accompanied by vegetable or cereal protein, e.g., pulses and oatmeal.

(7) Decide upon the protein ingredients of the meal first; next consider the protective materials such as the dairy foods, fruits and vegetables, and finally, supply energy foods such as bread, cereals, fats and sugar to satisfy appetite.

Let us now examine the following typical schedule of meals.

BREAKFAST

Porridge or other cereal, or fruit, with milk and sugar.

Bacon, or egg, or fish, or sausage, with fried potatoes or fried bread.

Bread with butter or margarine.

Marmalade or jam.

Tea or coffee. Cocoa or milk for children.

MID-MORNING SNACK

Adolescents and men and women doing heavy manual work should have a mid-morning snack consisting of body-building material such as cheese, eggs, meat or fish and a protective food in the form of fruit or raw vegetable, e.g., cheese and watercress sandwiches, sardine and parsley sandwiches, or meat pasty with tomatoes.

Milk for children and expectant and nursing mothers.

DINNER

Soup, if desired.

Meat or cheese or fish or eggs.

Potatoes.

Fresh vegetables (root or green or both).

Pudding or fruit with milk or custard.

Water to drink.

TEA

Main dish of cheese or fish or egg or meat.

Raw vegetable salad or fruit and cream or custard.

Bread and butter or margarine.

Cakes, pastry, scones or biscuits.

Jam, syrup or honey if desired.

Tea. Milk for children.

SUPPER

Hot milk and biscuits.

In addition, young children and expectant and nursing mothers should have orange juice before breakfast and cod liver oil after meals.

Plenty of water should be drunk daily.

Each of these meals will be found to contain body-building material, protective material and energy material. For example:

Breakfast

Body-building material. High biological value protein of milk, bacon, eggs, fish or sausage supplemented by the protein of oatmeal and bread.

Protective minerals and vitamins. Mainly from milk, butter, margarine, oatmeal, bread, bacon, egg and fish.

Energy material. Mainly from oatmeal, bread, sugar, marmalade and jam.

Mid-morning snack

Body-building material. High biological value protein from cheese, eggs, meat or fish, supplemented by protein of flour.

Protective material. From fruit or raw vegetables.

Dinner

Stimulation of appetite and flow of digestive juices from soup.

Body-building material. High biological value protein from milk or custard, meat, fish, cheese or eggs, supplemented by protein from vegetables and flour or cereal in pudding.

Protective minerals and vitamins. Mainly from meat, cheese, fish or eggs, potatoes, vegetables and milk (fresh or in custard).

Energy material. Mainly from potatoes, root vegetables, and cereals, fat and sugar in pudding and custard.

Tea

Body-building material. High biological value protein from cheese or fish or egg or meat supplemented by protein from flour of bread, cakes, scones, pastry, biscuits and so on.

Protective minerals and vitamins. Mainly from cheese, fish, egg or meat, raw vegetable or fruit, butter or margarine, bread and milk.

Energy material. Mainly from bread, butter or margarine, cakes, scones, pastry, biscuits and so on, jam, syrup or honey.

Supper

Body-building material. High biological value protein from milk supplemented by protein of flour.

Protective minerals and vitamins. From milk.

Energy material. From biscuits.

The additional calcium, vitamins A and D and vitamin C required by young children, expectant and nursing mothers will be supplied respectively by the extra milk, cod liver oil and orange juice they take.

THE FEEDING OF INFANTS AND YOUNG CHILDREN

There is no doubt that breast feeding is the best method of feeding a young baby. His mother's milk contains most of the materials he requires and in the correct proportions. If the mother is unable to breast-feed her baby he must be bottle-fed on specially prepared baby milks. These are dried milks which have been "humanised" by having their composition adjusted closely to that of human milk. The instructions for making up these powdered milks should be accurately followed and the correct amounts of liquid and powder must be used.

The baby will need additional protective materials and should be trained to take orange juice and cod liver oil from a spoon to supply vitamins C, A and D.

Having been taught to take liquids from a spoon the next stage is to teach the baby to take some solid food from a spoon. He can be gradually introduced to bread and other cereals, mashed potatoes, sieved green vegetables, mashed hard-boiled egg yolk, minced meat, particularly liver, and fish. When he reaches a weight of 5½ kg the use of fruits and vegetables should be extended and jam, treacle, dripping and butter added to the baby's diet. The sieved greens, egg yolk and minced liver are especially important, because milk contains very little iron and by this time the baby will have used up the supply of iron stored up in his liver at birth.

The period from one to two years of age is an important transition stage during which the young child should be taught to use his teeth by being made to chew ripe fruit, fairy toast and rusks. It is during this transition from a milk diet to a mixed solid diet that likes and dislikes and habits of diet are largely formed. These may persist throughout life and great care must be taken by the mother to inculcate a liking for the right kinds of food.

By the time he is three years of age the child should be ready and willing to eat any of the usual foods of an adult in, of course, smaller quantities and with a preponderance of protective mineral and vitamin foods and body-building proteins. Young children can only take small amounts of food at each meal and it is essential that all they eat is of high nutritive value. A half a litre of milk daily should still be the foundation of the diet along with cheese, butter, vitaminised margarine, fresh fruit and vegetables, and fat fish. Bread, toast, plain cake, biscuits, cereals, steamed puddings and jam should be the main energy suppliers.

THE FEEDING OF OLDER CHILDREN

From early childhood to adolescence the principles of diet remain the same but there is a gradual increase in the amounts required. Appetite can normally be relied upon to decide the amounts required but the mere satisfaction of appetite by the energy foods should never be allowed to take place at the expense of the body-building and protective foods.

During adolescence the appetites of both boys and girls increase enormously and should be satisfied but, again, not at the expense of the body-building and protective foods since growth of flesh and bone are very rapid at this stage. The iron-containing foods—green vegetables, eggs and liver—are especially important to girls during puberty and care should be taken to ensure their getting sufficient of them. The energy requirements of boys and girls between the ages of fourteen and twenty-one are greater than those of the average adult and can only be met by their receiving an increased amount of energy foods.

THE FEEDING OF ADULTS

The energy intake of adults should correspond to their energy output and will be higher for the manual than for the sedentary worker. The amount of protein recommended for the manual worker is higher than for a sedentary worker, as it is suggested that protein should provide 10–15% of the total energy intake, and so protein rises as kcal needs rise. In fact, manual work does *not* require extra protein and the British recommended intakes are a concession to our desire to have bigger protein portions with the larger energy food intake. This greater amount also increases the vitamins and minerals provided by the protein rich foods.

The extra energy needed by manual workers will be mainly provided by extra fat and carbohydrate foods and this increase must be accompanied by a corresponding increase in the consumption of vitamin B_1 (thiamine).

A woman's energy output is less than a man's and she normally requires less food. In the case of the protective foods, particularly the iron-containing foods, her needs are, however, almost certainly greater than those of a man. Many housewives make the mistake of ensuring an adequate diet for their husbands and children at the sacrifice of their own which all too frequently consists too largely of tea, bread, cakes and so on.

Expectant and nursing mothers should obviously pay special attention to their diets. The body-building and protective foods will need to be increased in amount. In addition to extra protein and vitamins there will be an increased need of calcium and iron. This increase in the body-building and protective foods should take place gradually from the earliest stages of pregnancy and not be concentrated into the last few months as is frequently done.

Expectant and nursing mothers should have a litre of milk daily and increased servings of green vegetables, fruit, particularly citrus fruit, eggs, as well as cod liver oil and orange juice. They should also drink a litre and a half of water daily. Extra carbohydrate should be avoided.

There is little scientific evidence respecting any special nutritional needs of old people. It is, however, reasonable to assume that their energy output will decrease with advancing age and their food requirements consequently diminish. Their digestive powers will almost certainly be less than they formerly were. Consequently old people should take food fairly frequently in small amounts at a time and in an easily digestible form.

There is no reliable evidence that old people require less protein than younger adults while their need for calcium, phosphorus and vitamin D will probably be as great as that of younger adults in view of their susceptibility to bone injury due to the gradual demineralisation which takes place in bones with advancing age. So far as the vitamins are concerned the most we can say is that since old people require less energy they will need less carbohydrates and consequently less of the B-vitamins. Vitamin C will probably be needed in as large amounts as by younger adults, particularly if the diet is restricted and monotonous as it frequently is in old age. Vitamins A and D will probably be needed in as large amounts as for younger adults.

It must be admitted that there is still a great deal to be learned about the nutritional needs of old people. There is no doubt, however, that a healthy old age is very largely a result of good nutrition in earlier life.

THE FEEDING OF INVALIDS AND CONVALESCENTS

The feeding of invalids and convalescents is an important factor in their recovery and should receive very careful attention.

In the case of certain diseases, such as diabetes, anaemia, scarlet fever and typhoid fever, the doctor will prescribe what the patient should eat and his instructions should be rigidly followed. Quite apart from such special cases the mere fact that the patient is no longer leading a normal active life will necessitate changes in diet whether or not the illness affects the digestive system.

In the early stages of diseases marked by a rise in temperature solid foods should not be given. Instead, a liquid diet consisting of milk and milk foods such as arrowroot and milk jelly or beef tea will be sufficient. When the patient's temperature is down to normal a light diet may be given. This should be of an easily digested nature and served in small quantities only. In addition to milk and milk foods, eggs in the form of custards, meat broths, white fish, citrus fruits, toast and biscuits may be given. During convalescence the diet becomes of the greatest importance. It should be increased in amount and should be such as to build up strength and wasted tissues especially after a long and wasting illness. The more easily digested protein foods such as milk, eggs, white fish and poultry are of the greatest value for this purpose unless any of them are forbidden by the doctor. These foods should be given in their most digestible form, e.g., fish steamed, meat stewed or minced, and eggs scrambled or coddled.

The diet of an invalid or convalescent should contain plenty of foods rich in vitamin C. This can be given in the form of fruit, especially oranges, lemons and grapefruits, and fresh green vegetables. One green vegetable cooked so as to preserve the maximum amount of vitamin C should be given daily along with potatoes. Whenever possible a serving of raw vegetable as a salad, in sandwiches or as a garnish to a hot dish should be included daily. If cooked or raw vegetables cannot be taken, the patient should be given the necessary daily dose of vitamin C in the form of rose-hip syrup, blackcurrant purée or concentrated orange juice.

Indigestible greasy foods should not be given at any stage of an illness. This precludes pork, ham, sausages, pastry, all fried foods, hot buttered toast. New bread, and highly flavoured sauces, pickles and spices are also unsuitable. Foods such as beef tea, meat extracts and jellies may help to stimulate the patient's appetite but it should always be realised that they have very little food value and should form only a minor part of the invalid's diet.

Patients are frequently finicky about their food and their appetites need to be tempted. This can be done by serving absolutely fresh food of the finest quality; by varying the food and the method of cooking as much as possible to avoid monotony; by serving small helpings in a dainty and attractive way since nothing is more likely to upset the patient's appetite than the sight of too much food badly served; by being punctual with meals and by never preparing food or leaving food behind in the sickroom.

The correct feeding of invalids and convalescents is frequently an arduous and trying task requiring both skill and patience but, once the patient is convalescent, carefully chosen food properly cooked can often do more than anything else to ensure a speedy recovery.

There are now available scientifically prepared powders, such as Metercal and Complan, which supply complete diets for invalids who cannot eat solid foods. They consist of a mixture of skimmed milk powder, soya bean flour, corn oil, minerals and vitamins and contain every essential nutrient. Flavourings are added to make the powders more palatable. The powders can be dissolved quickly and smoothly in water, hot or cold milk or both. Increasing amounts are being used as slimming diets.

VEGETARIAN DIET

Strictly speaking a vegetarian diet is one which is completely confined to food derived from plant life. Not only are meat, fish and poultry excluded but also milk, butter, eggs and cheese since these also are derived from animals. Such a diet is very limited in choice, monotonous, unattractive and very bulky. It is difficult to introduce much variety into meals consisting only of cereals, vegetables, fruits, nuts, honey, sugar and treacle. However, there are in the world a few races and religious sects which subsist upon such a diet. They include high caste Hindus and Trappist Monks. It is very doubtful if the human digestive system is adapted to the strictly vegetarian (sometimes called "vegan") diet.

Apart from its lack of variety such a diet presents great difficulty in supplying the body with the essential amino-acids more easily found in animal proteins, the fat-soluble vitamins A and D and the minerals, calcium, phosphorus and iron. The best sources of protein for the strict vegetarian are the legumes, peas, beans, lentils and soya, wheat, oats and nuts, but their proteins are not of such high biological value as those of animal foods nor are they as easily digested. The other plant foods—green vegetables, root vegetables, fruits, honey, sugar and treacle—are of little or no value as sources of proteins. Carbohydrate starch and sugar to supply energy would be easily provided in such a diet by the cereals, legumes, root vegetables, tubers, honey, sugar and treacle. Fat would mainly come from nuts and soya but large amounts would need to be eaten. Of the vitamins there would be no lack of vitamin C since such a large amount of fruit and vegetables would be consumed. The B-vitamins would also be well represented in the whole-grain cereals. Vitamin A, in the form of carotene, would be obtained from carrots, watercress, parsley, tomatoes and dark green vegetables but, again, large amounts would have to be eaten to meet the body's requirements, while vitamin D would be still more difficult to acquire. The important minerals, calcium, phosphorus and iron, would be difficult to supply in sufficient amounts since the legumes are the only plant foods supplying anything but negligible quantities. We are thus driven to the conclusion that the exclusive use of plant foods has no scientific justification.

Many so-called vegetarian diets include milk, butter, cheese and eggs. They are merely diets which do not include flesh foods. With these additions there is no difficulty in supplying the animal proteins, vitamins A and D and the minerals calcium, phosphorus and iron. The difficulty of introducing variety and attractiveness into meals would still remain but to a much smaller degree and the diet would not be so bulky. Nevertheless, great skill and care would be needed to ensure that the same foods are not served too frequently and the dishes do not become monotonous and uninteresting.

While the strictly vegetarian diet is cheaper than the normal mixed diet, the addition of milk, butter, cheese and eggs in the necessary quantities is apt to make the non-flesh diet rather expensive. There can be no doubt that the use of meat, fish and poultry makes the preparation of attractive, appetising meals much easier and the provision of the necessary nutrients more certain. As in the case of the strictly vegetarian diet, there is no scientific justification for the non-flesh diet for the normal healthy person.

SLIMMING

With increased medical knowledge it has become very evident that anybody who is grossly over-weight is abusing his body and is likely to die far sooner than he should. Gross fatness leads to physical laziness and so increases itself, but medical research has also revealed that some fat people have an inbuilt tendency to lay down carbohydrate as fat. There is also evidence that eating fulfils a psychological need with some people and that sugar addiction should be considered as seriously as addiction to tobacco.

In view of this evidence slimming becomes a medical necessity for some as well as a fashionable fad with others.

The aim of all slimming diets must be twofold. The first aim is to reduce weight; this can only be done by cutting the consumption of food and in particular of fats and carbohydrates. The second aim of any slimming diet should be to develop new, less fattening, eating habits so that once the diet has stopped the person does not return to a diet overloaded with the foods that had previously caused him to be fat.

Because one should develop new eating habits it is important that a slimming diet should be attractive and satisfying, and of course it must contain all the nutrients essential for health. A high protein diet is probably the easiest long-term diet as it allows a large consumption of meat and fish together with leafy vegetables and fruit. It is however, an expensive diet, and a cheaper method is to eliminate sugar and all fried foods as well as reducing the amount of all carbohydrate foods eaten.

Whatever diet is used care must be taken not to reduce the intake of vital nutrients to dangerous levels, and this is why it is advisable to seek qualified advice on any diet that is to be used for more than a few days.

ECONOMY IN DIET

True economy in diet means the provision of the necessary nutrients in adequate amounts at the lowest price, without, however, making the diet monotonous and unappetising. No matter how cheap it may be, no diet is really economical which does not supply the necessary kilocalories, protein, minerals and vitamins. On the other hand, the fact that a large amount of money is being spent on food does not necessarily guarantee a sound diet.

The cheapest sources of animal proteins are cheese and herrings. The cheapest sources of energy are bread and margarine. Such a combination would also supply calcium, phosphorus, vitamin A and, if the bread be made from fortified flour, some iron and B-vitamins. It would be lacking in vitamin C which could be most cheaply provided by cabbage, and vitamin D which could be cheaply supplied by a teaspoonful of cod liver oil. Theoretically, at any rate, it would be possible to subsist on such a diet but even the poorest person in the land would quickly tire of its monotony. Obviously, variety would have to be introduced and it is here that the diet can easily become uneconomical.

Meat and white fish are more expensive body-building foods than cheese and herrings which provide valuable calcium, phosphorus and vitamin A and energy in addition to animal proteins. Milk is a relatively dear food but is indispensable on account of its body-building and protective materials. Salmon and sardines are excellent foods but the same proteins, calcium, phosphorus, iodine, vitamins A and D can be more cheaply provided by herrings. Bacon is an economical body-building food because it supplies energy as well as proteins. Eggs, in spite of their calcium, phosphorus, iron, vitamins A and D are, unfortunately, dear sources of proteins and kilocalories.

Some new proteins are coming on to the market. Most of them at the moment are made from soya beans, but foods from bacterial, yeast and fungal sources will soon follow. These foods offer cheap sources of protein and if supplemented with other nutrients will become useful and economical additions to our range of foods.

The greatest economy in diet can be made in the carbohydrate energy foods since they form the largest part of the diet and show the greatest variations in price. The cereals, potatoes, pulses and dried fruits are the cheapest of the carbohydrate foods. Sugar is a cheap energy food but supplies nothing else.

Green vegetables and fresh fruits must be judged as sources of vitamin C and minerals and the cabbage is easily the cheapest, followed by tomatoes and oranges. All green vegetables and fresh fruits are dear for kilocalories but their vitamins and minerals make them indispensable.

To sum up we may say that the diet may be made more economical but no less nutritionally satisfactory by an increased use of cheese, herrings, vitaminised margarine, whole-grain cereals, potatoes, pulses and dried fruits. Milk, green vegetables and fresh fruit are essential and it is unwise to economise in their use in spite of their relatively high cost. To be economical the amounts of meat, white fish and eggs in the diet should be reduced.

22 The Digestion, Absorption and Metabolism of Food

DIGESTION

We have seen that food supplies the body with heat and energy, with material for growth and repair, and with substances which regulate the mechanism of the body. With very few exceptions, foods as eaten are not in a suitable form to be utilised by the body for any of these purposes. The majority of foods must be broken down into simple soluble substances before they can be absorbed into the body through the walls of the digestive tract. It is only then that the body can utilise them. This breakdown process is carried out by the mechanical action of the teeth and other parts of the digestive tract but chiefly by the chemical action of various digestive juices. The whole breakdown process is known as *digestion*.

ENZYMES

Enzymes are protein catalysts; in other words, they are proteins which speed reactions but remain unchanged themselves at the end of the reaction.

All enzymes have a name ending in "ase." Thus a protein-splitting enzyme is a *protease*; a fat or "lipoid" splitting enzyme is a *lipase*; and one which breaks starch is an *amylase* (from the latin for starch).

Some enzymes were named before the agreement on the "ase" ending and these names may still be used in some books.

Certain enzymes cannot work unless another particular chemical is present. This second substance is called the *co-enzyme*.

Enzymes are very sensitive to temperature changes and to the degree of acidity or alkalinity; their activity will be prevented by incorrect conditions.

THE DIGESTIVE TRACT

The digestive tract, or alimentary canal, consists essentially of a long tube open at both ends, the mouth and the anus. Although this tube passes through the body it is, in a sense, external to it and while food remains in this tube or "gut" it is really outside the body. It is only when food passes through the walls of the gut into the blood stream that it has actually passed into the body.

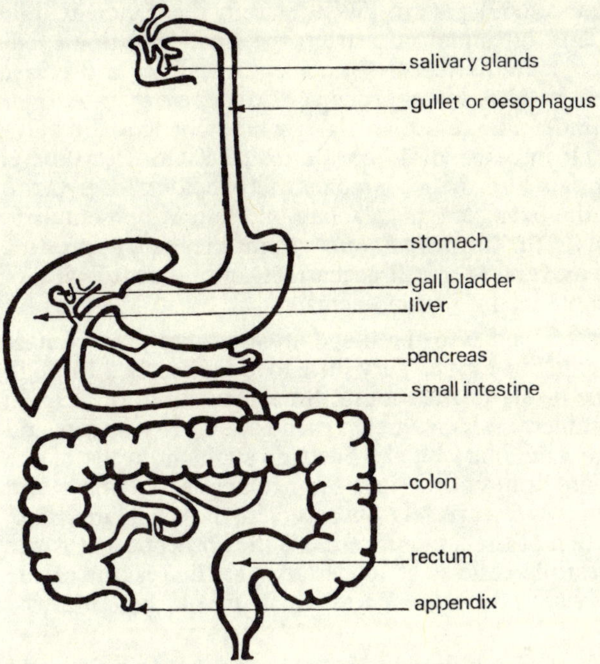

The digestive system.

The main parts of the digestive tract are the mouth, gullet, stomach, small intestine and large intestine. In the adult, the small intestine is about 6 metres long and the large intestine about 2 metres in length. Various glands, such as the salivary glands of the mouth, the gastric glands of the stomach, the liver and pancreas, secrete digestive juices into the gut which break down the food by chemical action into simpler and soluble substances which can be absorbed into the blood.

The digestion of food is carried out in stages in separate parts of the digestive tract—the mouth, stomach and intestines—by digestive juices containing specialised enzymes. In the mouth, the salivary glands secrete saliva containing an amylase which converts starch into soluble forms of carbohydrate. In the stomach, the gastric glands secrete gastric juice containing a protease (pepsin), which, in the presence of hydrochloric acid, converts proteins into simpler substances known as peptones. In the small intestine, food comes into contact with pancreatic juice from the pancreas, bile from the liver and intestinal juice from the small intestine itself. Pancreatic juice contains three distinct enzymes: (*a*) a protease (trypsin) which breaks down proteins and peptones into their constituent amino-acids, (*b*) an amylase, which changes the polysaccharide starch into the disaccharide maltose and (*c*) a lipase, which splits up fats into their component fatty acids and glycerol. The bile from the liver contains alkaline bile salts which emulsify fats. Enzymes in the intestinal juice from the small intestine complete the conversion of disaccharides into glucose and of proteins and peptones into amino-acids.

The absorption of food into the blood stream takes place almost entirely in the small intestine. Very little food is absorbed through the lining of the inside of the mouth. Small quantities of alcohol, sugar, soluble mineral salts, soluble vitamins, i.e., B-vitamins and vitamin C, and water may be absorbed through the walls of the stomach. Carbohydrates, proteins, fats, minerals, vitamins and water are practically completely absorbed in the small intestine. The main function of the large intestine is the absorption of water from the indigestible residue of foodstuffs and the residue of the digestive juices which form the faeces which are passed out of the body.

Such, briefly, is the sequence of the processes of digestion and absorption which will now be considered in greater detail.

Digestion in the mouth

The process of reducing food to physical and chemical states suitable for absorption is started in the mouth. During mastication the teeth cut and grind the food to a small size and the tongue and the mouth muscles by their movements mix up the food with the saliva secreted by the salivary glands. The act of mastication stimulates the salivary glands but the secretion of saliva is more of a reflex action in response to the stimulus of taste and, to a less extent, of smell. Salivation is also closely linked with the emotions. The mere thought of food, particularly when one is hungry, is often sufficient to "make the mouth water." On the other hand, fear, excitement or worry may stop secretion. Pleasant surroundings, good company and cheerful conversation are all conducive to increased flow of saliva and hence to improved digestion.

Saliva acts as a moistener and lubricator so as to allow the soft bolus of food to pass easily down the gullet or oesophagus. The amylase has the power of converting starch into maltose and dextrin but only when the solution is neutral or slightly alkaline and when the cellulose covering of the starch grains has been broken open by cooking. The majority of people, instead of chewing their food properly, swallow it almost as quickly as eaten and the amylase has practically no opportunity of effecting any chemical change in the mouth. The action of the amylase, however, continues for a time in the stomach until the hydrochloric acid of the stomach acidifies the food. When starch grains are cooked with fat, as in pastry, fried potatoes or batter, the digestive action of the amylase is considerably hindered and indigestion may be experienced.

Digestion in the stomach

The chief purpose of the stomach is not really as a digestive organ but as a reservoir dealing out its contents in conveniently manageable quantities to the first part of the small intestine—the duodenum. Another useful function is to bring foods of different temperatures all to the temperature of the body (36·9° C) and to melt fats. The stomach's extraordinarily rich supply of blood-vessels makes it well adapted to these purposes.

The mechanical action of the powerful muscles in the walls of the stomach churns the food and serves to bring the food into close contact with the gastric juice and reduce it to a more liquid consistency as "chyme."

The stimulation of the flow of gastric juice in readiness for the digestion of protein foods depends partly upon the chemical nature of the food passing into the stomach and partly upon psychological factors. The dextrin produced by the partial digestion of starch in the mouth and the water in the saliva both excite the gastric glands. Hence the justification for the nibbling at a roll before taking soup. The extractives of meat, especially as concentrated in several proprietary articles, are powerful stimulants of the gastric glands. Ordinary soups act in the same manner; hence their place at the beginning of the ordinary dinner menu. The psychological factors of smell, sound and sight, and so on, which promote the flow of saliva also increase the flow of gastric juice. The flow is checked by worry, excitement or anger, and digestion thus hindered.

The hydrochloric acid secreted in the stomach acts as a powerful antiseptic: a fact doubtless of great importance in the case of the chance raw food of the savage, and not wholly without significance in the food of civilised man.

The protease of the gastric juice, in association with hydrochloric acid, brings about a certain amount of digestion of proteins into peptones. Its main purpose, however, is probably to produce such semi-digested substances as will stimulate the secretion of further enzymes required for fuller digestion in the succeeding portion of the gut—the duodenum. The gastric juice of children also contains a protease enzyme (rennin), which curdles milk in readiness for digestion in the small intestine.

Digestion in the small intestine

Chyme, on becoming thoroughly impregnated with the acid gastric juice, causes the valve (pylorus) between the stomach and the first

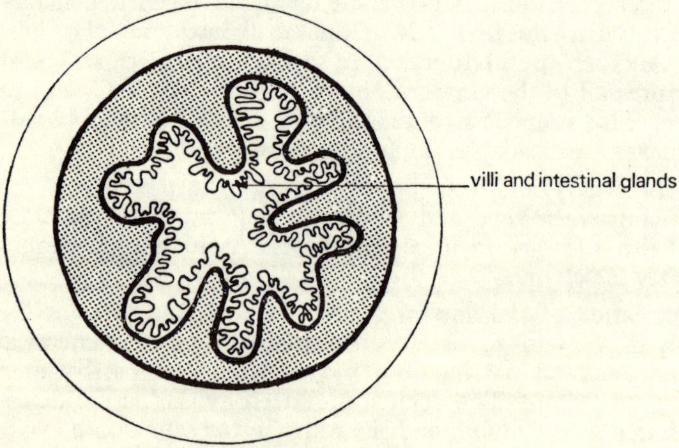

Cross-section of small intestine (much magnified).

portion of the small intestine to relax and, in small quantities at a time, it passes into the duodenum.

The reaction of the small intestine is alkaline and one of the first results of the admission of acid is the stimulation of the flow of pancreatic juice from the pancreas and the flow of bile from the liver. The bile juice contains bile salts which emulsify the fats and increase the activity of the pancreatic lipase.

The pancreatic juice contains proteases which change proteins and peptones to amino-acids; an amylase which continues the work of the salivary amylase breaking the starch into disaccharides and lipase which breaks up some of the emulsified fat into fatty acids and glycerol.

As the food passes further down the small intestine it has poured on to it an intestinal juice which contains several enzymes and is made by glands present in the lining of the small intestine.

The final breakdown of proteins into amino-acids is brought about by proteases in the intestinal juice. The intestinal juice also contains maltase which converts maltose to glucose, sucrase (or invertase) which converts sucrose to glucose and fructose, and lactase which converts lactose to glucose and galactose.

Thus, as the food, or chyle as it is now called, is moved along the length of the small intestine by the peristaltic action of its muscles,

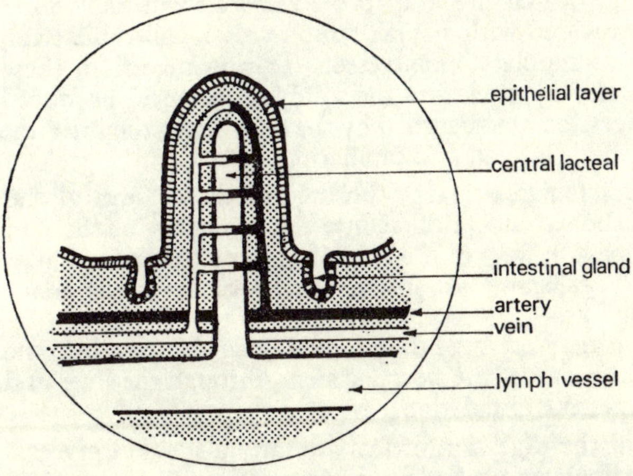

Section through wall of small intestine (much magnified).

all of it that is digestible is converted into simple and soluble substances which can pass through into the surrounding blood capillaries and lacteals to be utilised by the body.

Digestion in the large intestine

The large intestine contains no digestive juices but is rich in bacteria. By the time the mass reaches it all the digestible food has been absorbed. The material left is largely cellulose which is indigestible in man, the residue of digestive juices and bacteria. Water is absorbed from it all along the large intestine so that it reaches the rectum in a semi-solid or solid form. This more or less solid consistency exerts a pressure on the muscles of the rectum which leads to its expulsion from the body as faeces.

The bacteria in the large intestine produce certain of the B-group of vitamins and, to a small extent, supplement the body's supply.

ABSORPTION

Absorption is the term applied to the passage of the products of digestion through the walls of the digestive tract. The small intestine is the part of the digestive tract through which practically the whole of the absorption of foods into the blood-stream takes place. The mucous membrane lining of the small intestine is especially adapted for the purpose by being thrown into permanent folds throughout which are tiny projections known as "villi." Each villus is provided with a small lymph vessel, called a lacteal, and a network of capillary bloodvessels. During digestion, these villi are surrounded by chyle and the soluble substances produced as a result of digestion are absorbed by the cells lining the intestine and are passed to the lacteals and capillaries.

Monosaccharides (single sugars), the final digestive form of the various food carbohydrates, diffuse into the capillaries of the villi and ultimately pass by way of the portal vein into the liver. There any fructose or galactose are converted to glucose, the main monosaccharide.

The amino-acids derived from the protein foods also pass into the capillaries and, by way of the portal system, through the liver and thence into the general circulation.

The products of the digestion of fats are fatty acids and glycerol as well as some finely emulsified undissociated fats. The fatty acids and glycerol pass into the intestinal cells. There the free fatty acids are combined in the cell with glycerol present in the cell to form fats. The glycerol split off from the original fat is metabolised on its own, passing into the portal vein and thence to the liver where it is available for the production of energy. The fats pass into the lacteals, the lymphatic and thoracic ducts, which open into the main vein just before the right auricle of the heart.

METABOLISM

Metabolism is the term used for the many different chemical processes which take place in the tissues and cells of the body. Distinction is commonly made between those concerned with the building up of the various substances provided by food into the substances characteristic of the tissues and cells (anabolism), and those concerned with the liberation of energy and the production of final breakdown waste products such as carbon dioxide, water and urea (catabolism).

Glucose is normally found in the blood in fairly steady concentration. It is the more immediate supply of energy for cells and tissues. Used-up glucose is quickly replaced by the conversion of the stored carbohydrate, glycogen, in the liver being changed into glucose. The liberation of the available energy of this "blood sugar" is a complicated process, involving the absorption of oxygen from the blood-stream and the liberation of carbon dioxide and water as breakdown waste products. The energy appears in various forms; as heat, as muscular work and as chemical energy in a great variety of compounds associated with the living stuff of cells and tissues.

Glucose absorbed in excess of body requirements is stored in the liver and muscles as animal starch (glycogen) or, when reduced to fat, is retained as depot fat throughout the body, but chiefly in the abdomen. This reserve food supply can be drawn upon when required, being first re-converted into glucose by partial oxidation.

The hormone insulin manufactured in the pancreas controls the blood sugar level.

The complete oxidation of fat in the body is a more difficult process than that of glucose. When completely oxidised, fat yields simply carbon dioxide and water, but incomplete oxidation results in the formation of ketones which give rise to ketosis or biliousness.

This condition can usually be relieved by adding sugar to the diet and largely prevented by a diet in which fats are well balanced by carbohydrates. Excess fat is stored in the fat depots around the body.

The essential compounds for the building up of the many different cell proteins are the amino-acids. These are taken in the necessary amount and variety from the blood-stream so that the cells and tissues can grow and develop and wastage be made good. Amino-acids available to the body in the food which are in excess of the body's needs or are unwanted, are carried to the liver where they are disintegrated into carbohydrate or fat residues and nitrogen residues. The nitrogen residues are ultimately excreted from the system as urea, or similar substances, in urine. The carbohydrate residues are available for the production of heat and energy. The use of excess protein as fuel instead of as building and repair substance is uneconomic. Wastage of protein in this manner can be largely avoided by the practice of mixed carbohydrate and protein meals.

SUMMARIES

Digestion

(a) In the Mouth (Alkaline)
(1) Food broken up, moistened and lubricated.
(2) A small amount of cooked starch changed into maltose.

(b) In the Stomach (Acid)
(1) More mixing and mechanical breakdown of food.
(2) For a time, more cooked starch changed into maltose.
(3) Conversion of proteins into peptones started.
(4) Milk is curdled by the hydrochloric acid.
(5) In children milk is clotted.

(c) In the Small Intestine (Alkaline)
(1) Carbohydrates converted to monosaccharides.
(2) Proteins and peptones converted into amino-acids.
(3) Fats emulsified and split into fatty acids and glycerol.

(d) In the Large Intestine
Some of the B-vitamins formed.

Nutrients

(a) Carbohydrates

(i) Sugars

(1) Unchanged in mouth and stomach.

(2) In small intestine, enzymes convert each type of sugar into monosaccharides.

(ii) Starch

(1) Enzyme, amylase, in saliva begins conversion of starch into maltose in the mouth.

(2) Remaining starch converted into maltose in small intestine by action of pancreatic amylase and finally into glucose by intestinal maltose.

(b) Fats

(1) Unchanged in mouth and stomach.

(2) Emulsified by bile in small intestine.

(3) Split into fatty acids and glycerol by lipase of pancreatic juice in small intestine.

(c) Proteins

(1) Unchanged in the mouth.

(2) Protease of gastric juice begins conversion of proteins into peptones in the stomach.

(3) Conversion of proteins into peptones and peptones into amino-acids by enzymes of pancreatic juice and intestinal juice completed in the small intestine.

(d) Minerals

(1) Soluble salts of sodium and potassium are rapidly absorbed in stomach and small intestine. Excess is eliminated by kidneys in urine.

(2) Calcium absorbed in small intestine. Unavailable calcium passes through large intestine in faeces.

(3) Amounts of iron required by the body absorbed through small intestine. Excess iron is passed out of body in faeces.

(e) Vitamins

(i) Water soluble vitamins (B and C).

(1) Absorbed in stomach and small intestine.

(2) Excess cannot be stored in the body and is eliminated by the kidneys in urine.

(ii) Fat-soluble vitamins (A and D).
(1) Absorbed only in small intestine.
(2) Excess can be stored in the liver.

Absorption

(a) In the Mouth
Very little.

(b) In the Stomach
Small quantities of alcohol, sugar, soluble mineral salts and soluble vitamins (B and C) and water.

(c) In the Small Intestine
Practically the whole of the absorption of carbohydrates, proteins, fats, minerals, vitamins and water.

(d) In the Large Intestine
Water and some B-vitamins.

Metabolism

(a) Carbohydrates
(1) Glucose oxidised to carbon dioxide and water with production of heat and energy.
(2) Excess glucose stored as glycogen or fat.

(b) Fats
(1) Oxidised to carbon dioxide and water with production of heat and energy.
(2) Stored in the body's fat depots.

(c) Proteins
(1) Amino-acids used by tissues for building and repair.
(2) Oxidised for production of heat and energy.

Digestive juices

Juice	*Enzyme*	*Action*
Saliva	Amylase	Starch into maltose
Gastric juice	Protease (hydrochloric acid)	Proteins into peptones
Bile	(Alkaline salts)	Fats emulsified

Juice	*Enzyme*	*Action*
Pancreatic	(a) Protease	Proteins and peptones into amino-acids
	(b) Amylase	Starch and maltose into glucose
	(c) Lipase	Fats into fatty acids and glycerol
Intestinal	(a) Protease	Peptones into amino-acids
	(b) Maltase Lactase Sucrase	Disaccharides (maltose, lactose, cane sugar) to glucose, fructose and galactose.

INDEX

by Lilian Rubin, M.A.